MW01264464

CLINICAL ASSESSMENT
OF
NUTRITIONAL STATUS
A WORKING MANUAL

SECOND EDITION

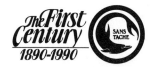

CLINICAL ASSESSMENT OF NUTRITIONAL STATUS
A WORKING MANUAL

SECOND EDITION

Alan H. Pressman
M.S., D.C., D.A.C.B.N., C.C.S.P., F.I.C.C.

President, Council on Nutrition
American Chiropractic Association

Adjunct Professor of Biology
College of Health Sciences
University of Bridgeport
Bridgeport, Connecticut

Formerly, Chairman, Department of Clinical Nutrition
New York Chiropractic College
New York, New York

Alan H. Adams
B.S., M.T., D.C., D.A.C.B.N.

Vice President, Chiropractic Education
Los Angeles College of Chiropractic
Whittier, California

Academic Dean
Canadian Memorial Chiropractic College

Director of Research
Council on Nutrition
American Chiropractic Association

Editorial Consultant
Journal of Manipulative and Physiological Therapeutics

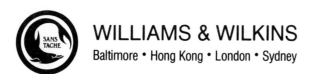

WILLIAMS & WILKINS
Baltimore • Hong Kong • London • Sydney

Editor: Jonathan W. Pine, Jr.
Associate Editor: Linda Napora
Copy Editor: Susan Vaupel
Designer: JoAnne Janowiak
Illustration Planner: Ray Lowman
Production Coordinator: Adèle Boyd

Accurate indications, adverse reactions, and dosage schedules for drugs are provided in this book, but it is possible that they may change. The reader is urged to review the package information data of the manufacturers of the medications mentioned.

Printed in the United States of America

First Edition 1982

Library of Congress Cataloging-in-Publication Data

Pressman, Alan H.
    Clinical assessment of nutritional status: a working manual /
Alan H. Pressman, Alan H. Adams.—2nd ed.
        p.   cm.
    Includes bibliographical references.
    ISBN 0-683-06970-5
    1. Nutrition—Evaluation. I. Adams, Alan H. II. Title.
    [DNLM: 1. Nutrition Disorders—diagnosis. 2. Nutritional Status.
WD 100 F936c]
RC621.P74   1990
616.3'9075—dc20
DNLM/DLC
for Library of Congress   89-24859
                                                                   CIP

90 91 92 93 94
1 2 3 4 5 6 7 8 9 10

PREFACE

The assessment of nutritional status has become an integral part of the total clinical evaluation—and eventual treatment program—undertaken with today's patient. It is the first and foremost step in the evaluation of nutritional needs and dietary deficiencies, and if properly performed and acted upon, the assessment is crucial to the prevention of future ill health. This second edition of *Clinical Assessment of Nutritional Status* provides an orderly series of guidelines, questions, tables, and forms to help practitioners make a scientific assessment of their patients' nutritional status. The information obtained can then be used to develop a successful intervention plan when such action is warranted.

Determined by comparing actual nutrient intake with overall nutrient need, nutritional status is a measure of malnutrition. Nutritional status includes disorders of both undernutrition and overnutrition, and it is assessed by examining a patient's personal history, dietary intake, body composition, tissue function, and metabolic activity. The unique anthropometric, biochemical, clinical, dietary, and physical data that result are then evaluated against established criteria in order to identify patients in need of further examination—as well as the subsequent treatment that they may require.

Generally, malnutrition or an unsatisfactory nutritional status is associated with enhanced morbidity and increased mortality. More specifically, it is linked to diminished growth and development, decreased physical and emotional strength, and a lessened ability to resist and fight disease. It also is tied to lengthier hospital stays and reduced organ functions.

Identifying a patient with nutritional deficiencies, then, is of paramount concern to the modern practitioner. Diagnosing someone who is obviously malnourished and already is suffering from various anatomical or functional limitations requires few special skills. But since the eventual consequences of poor nutritional status may be irreversible and even life threatening, it is critical that such patients be identified as early as possible. A logical and comprehensive procedure for nutritional assessment is expedient (see Nutritional Care Procedure for Intervention, p. viii).

The tools and techniques utilized in such an assessment must be diverse—and sensitive enough—to evaluate all of the many components that affect a patient's nutritional status. These include inadequate intake, inadequate absorption, defective utilization, and increased excretion. Clues to their presence can be found in the individual's physical appearance, health and social history, dietary habits, body composition, anthropometric constitution, and biochemical condition. Clues also come from special conditions such as pregnancy, obesity, athletic performance, and hospitalization. Information gathered in each of these areas will help the practitioner anticipate developing nutritional problems and outline the appropriate corrective measures.

Not every patient should undergo a comprehensive nutritional assessment, of course, but initial screenings can help identify those who are candidates for additional evaluation and potential intervention. While overt danger signals such as chronic alcoholism and gross weight problems should signify that a complete

**Nutritional Care
Procedure for Intervention**

Factors for the health care group
    Prevention
    Treatment
    Rehabilitation
    Maintenance

Six-step procedure
1. Identification
    Determine need for nutritional
      intervention
    Who is at risk?
2. Evaluation of nutritional status
    History
    Physical examination
    Anthropometrics
    Laboratory
    Dietary evaluation
3. Planning
    Objectives and goals
    Priorities

4. Implementation
    Dietary outline
    Menu planning
    Supplementation
    Life-style changes
    Support systems
5. Evaluation
    Results of treatment
    Changes of nutritional status
    Revisions as necessary
6. Monitoring
    Periodic reevaluations
    Future planning
    Reassessment of needs

assessment is in order, other more subtle symptoms also may indicate that a total examination is warranted.

Does the patient complain about gastrointestinal disorders, for example? Has there been prolonged use of oral contraceptives? Is there evidence of a lactase deficiency or a chronic disease state? Has the patient participated in a fad diet or been eating more in restaurants than at home? Was there any recent major surgery, illness, or injury? Has the patient been using large amounts of catabolic steroids, immunosuppressants, antibiotics, or anticonvulsant drugs? Is there evidence of mental illness?

The practitioner uses a variety of tools and techniques to appraise these factors and analyze their impact on nutritional status. Full medical and social histories, followed by a complete physical examination, are essential first steps. A comprehensive dietary evaluation, as well as specific laboratory procedures, also may be necessary. A variety of devices—from manual measuring tapes and skinfold calipers to computerized body composition and dietary data analyzers—assist in the process.

These tools and techniques supply the practitioner with the nutritional assessment data—the first step in providing patients with total nutritional care. The six-step model for nutritional intervention above demonstrates just how important such an initial identification is to the entire process.

Total nutritional management includes clinical and dietary investigation, determination of the problem, introduction of corrective measures, evaluation of progress, and monitoring any changing conditions that might require adjustments. The process, however, begins with the assessment of a patient's nutritional status. Information contained in the following pages will provide the practitioner with the core of facts that facilitate determination of nutritional status and thus the potential for its enhancement.

ACKNOWLEDGMENTS

The authors wish to thank Lewis A. Goodman for producing and packaging this volume, another in the series of Lewis A. Goodman Books.

In addition, the authors thank Howard Rothman for his invaluable help in the writing and preparation of this text.

CONTENTS

1

Case History and Physical Examination

The clinical assessment of nutritional status is a multi-faceted but orderly process that is undertaken along a well-marked path that is easily followed by the practitioner. Where this path ends only can be determined by traveling its entire route. It always begins, however, at the same point: with the case history and the physical examination.

In order to accurately determine the nutritional status of any patient, complete background data first must be obtained. This is derived from a comprehensive health, social, and family history, combined with an appraisal of the patient's relevant lifestyle peculiarities, psychological status, and eating patterns. (An accompanying dietary history, also of critical importance at this stage of the evaluation, is discussed in depth in Chapter 2.)

After these data are gathered, the next integral step in a nutritional analysis is the physical examination. Any abnormalities noted can be correlated with appropriate nutritional problems—even though this may be difficult because clinical signs of malnutrition often are mild, nonspecific, and the result of deficiencies in several nutrients. In addition, nonnutritional factors also play a role in the development of many physical problems. A complete examination, then, may take a considerable amount of time before the practitioner is able to pinpoint an abnormality as it relates to the patient's nutritional status.

With all of the above information in hand, the clinician is capable of creating an accurate, multidimensional picture of the patient in his or her own environment. This permits authoritative assessment of those areas in need of alteration; it also reveals those areas most capable of change, as well as those presenting resistance on the patient's part.

Health History

A Personal History Form (Fig. 1.1) should be distributed to all new patients as soon as they arrive, along with instructions to answer all questions before they leave the waiting area. This, along with a Nutritional Assessment Summary Form (Fig. 1.2)—to be completed by the clinician as pertinent information is revealed—will form the initial basis of the assessment.

PERSONAL HISTORY FORM

Date_____ Chart No._____

Name_____ Sex _____ Age_____

Occupation _____ Ethnic Background_____

Education_____ Marital Status_____

Family Group (# Members)_____

Present Weight _____ Height_____

Maximum Weight _____ Age at Maximum Weight_____

Desired Weight _____

Food Dislikes _____

Food Preferences _____

Foods Avoided for Health Reasons _____

Food Allergies _____

Food Cravings _____

Location Where You Eat Meals

    Breakfast _____Lunch_____Dinner_____

How many meals per week are eaten out? _____

Number of business or social activities involving food per week_____

_____

Number of meals eaten regularly:

    Each Day _____ Number on Weekends_____

Number of snacks eaten per day_____

Number on Weekends_____

Where do food supplies come from:

    _____ Store _____ Home Produced _____ Home Preserved

What food supplies are home produced and preserved: _____

_____

_____

Are facilities for cooking and storage adequate? _____

    _____ Oven _____ Refrigerator _____ Freezer _____ Blender

                                               Food Grinder

    _____ Range Top, Hot Plate, Electric Fry Pan _____ Other

For how many people do you cook?_____

Figure 1.1. Personal History Form. By using a form such as this, the clinician is able to keep track of the patient's usual dietary and exercise habits.

The Major Complaint

It is the practitioner's responsibility to determine and investigate the patient's presenting complaint. The problem must be thoroughly examined as it relates to either under- or over-nutrition. Once the major complaint is evaluated and can be traced to its primary cause, the case history then can be used to help refine and modify the diagnosis. Once the patient is seen in the examining room, a complete history of the presenting problem should be gathered.

Source of meals_____(Self)   _____(Others)

Size of meal portion: Small _____   Moderate _____

Large _____   Extra Large _____

Frequency of: Frying _____   Baking _____   Boiling _____

Cups of coffee or tea per day_____

With sugar _____   Cream _____   Milk _____

Soft drink use: Daily _____   Weekends _____

Diet _____   Regular _____

Alcohol use: Daily _____   Beer _____   Wine

Hard Liquor _____

Weekends _____   Beer _____   Wine _____

Hard Liquor _____

Daily use of: Milk _____ Butter _____ Cream _____

Salt _____   Animal Fats _____   Fatty Meats _____

Eggs _____   Starch _____   Fruits _____

Vegetables _____   Desserts _____

Sweets _____   Chewing Gum _____

Breath Mints _____

Have you been on any of the following diets during the past year? Yes _____   No _____

Weight Loss _____   Diabetic _____   Low Salt (Sodium) _____

Low Fat _____   High Protein _____   Low Carbohydrate_____

High Fiber _____   Other _____

Are you a vegetarian? _____

Do you eat: _____ Eggs   _____ Milk   _____ Cheese, Yogurt

_____ Fish   _____ Chicken/Turkey

Work activity level:

_____ Sedentary   _____ Light Work   _____ Moderately Heavy

_____ Heavy Work

Do you take vitamin or mineral supplements? Yes_____   No_____

What kind _____ Dosage/day _____

_____   _____

_____   _____

_____   _____

_____   _____

Necessary information to be obtained includes:

Date of onset of symptoms
Severity of symptoms
Remission of symptoms
Treatment to relieve the problem
Any changes due to treatment
Patterns of weight gain or loss
Whether the body weight is 20% over or under the ideal
Any recent gain or loss of weight

NUTRITIONAL ASSESSMENT SUMMARY FORM

Name _____ Age _____ Sex _____

Case No. _____

Health History (including drug history):

_____

_____

_____

_____

Diet History (including recall and frequency survey):

_____

_____

_____

_____

Physical Examination (including anthropometric evaluation):

_____

_____

_____

_____

Laboratory Evaluation:

_____

_____

_____

_____

Summary and Impression:

_____

_____

_____

Figure 1.2.   Nutritional Assessment Summary Form. The results of a patient's health history, dietary history, physical examination and laboratory evaluation can be tracked— along with summaries and impressions—on a single form.

Are there any increased metabolic needs due to:

Injury
Infection
Burns
Hyperthyroidism
Trauma
Fever
Chronic illness
Degenerative disease
Protein-calorie malnutrition
Recent surgery

Preoperative status
Pregnancy
Lactation
Infancy
Adolescent growth spurt

Are there any increased nutrient losses due to:

Open wounds
Chronic blood loss
Draining abscesses
Draining fistula
Effusions
Exudative enteropathies
Renal dialysis
Protracted diarrhea
Vomiting

When and for how long have any of these conditions been present?

Coronary artery disease
Atherosclerosis-hyperlipodemia
Hypertension/hypotension
Stroke
Hypoglycemia
Diabetes
Malabsorption
Carcinoma
Chronic lung disease
Chronic infections
Chronic liver disease
Obesity
Anorexia
Anemia
Hepatitis
Asthma
Hives, eczema
Colitis
Peptic ulcer
Rheumatoid arthritis
Cancer
Ascites, edema
Parkinson's disease
Multiple sclerosis
Huntington's disease
Epilepsy
Spinal problems
   Scoliosis
   Disc problems
   Spinal dysfunction
Migraine headaches
Hyperthyroidism/hypothyroidism
Hypoadrenalism
Genitourinary problems
   Female:

> Amenorrhea
> Excessive bleeding
> Miscarriages
> Male:
>> Prostate
>> Urinary problems
> Hypogeusia/Hyposmia

Does the patient have any of these emotional problems:

Excessive stress
Anxiety
Depression
Anhedonia
Alcoholism/drug abuse
Nervous breakdown
Schizophrenia
Hyperactivity (in children)

Are any of these diseases of the gastrointestinal tract present:

Pancreatic insufficiency
Gallbladder disease
Congenital malformations
Malabsorption syndromes (celiac disease, parasites, Crohn's disease)
Diverticular disease
Partial or total gastrointestinal obstruction
Difficulty chewing or swallowing
Glossitis, stomitis, or esophagitis
Severe diarrhea or constipation
Lack of intrinsic factor
Blind-loop syndrome
Pernicious anemia

Has been any recent use of large doses of the following:

Antidepressants
Tranquilizers
Antitumor agents
Oral contraceptives
Steroids
Immunosuppressants
Anticonvulsants
Aspirin
Vitamins
Illegal drugs
  Marijuana
  Cocaine
  Hallucinogens
  Heroin

Is the patient allergic to any of the following:

Penicillin
Sulfa drugs
Aspirin

Codeine
Morphine
Antitoxins
Any foods

Additional questions to ask:

What kind of surgery has the patient had, and when?
What kind of x-rays? What areas of the body and when?
Has the patient taken nothing by mouth for 3 days or more?
Is there lactose intolerance or limited food preference?
Is the patient able to perform regular daily activities?
Are there any respiratory or genitourinary complaints?

Social History

The formation of a complete, composite picture is further aided through a full examination of the patient's family and ethnic background, medical history, present life situation, and factors that are motivating change. Some patients suffer from malnutrition, for example, because they are unable to purchase adequate food supplies; the dietary habits of others are affected because they either live alone or have problems with mobility. Thorough knowledge of the patient's social situation, therefore, will enable the clinician to identify and accentuate the positive aspects that will enhance health-producing dietary and lifestyle adjustments.

Familial History

It is important to ascertain the health status of all members of the patient's immediate family, as well as any diseases from which they may suffer (Fig. 1.3).

Ethnic Composition

Every ethnic group is susceptible to different degenerative diseases, and the practitioner must take great care to analyze the relevant factors applicable to each. Some examples are: Blacks—high blood pressure, atherosclerosis; Jews—diabetes, coronary artery disease; Northern Europeans—pernicious anemia.

Social History of the Patient

The following must be determined if it is not already known:

Age
Sex
Marital status
Number of children
Occupation
Educational level
Is income adequate for food?
Eats more than half of meals away from home?
Eats alone? With others?
Adequate food to combat psychological stress?

FAMILY HISTORY FORM

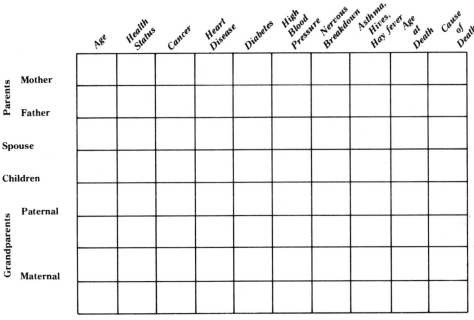

Figure 1.3.   Family History Form. The relevant health history of immediate family members can be tracked on a form and later aid the clinician in diagnosing the patient.

Life Events Indicator

Life events as indicators of potential degenerative disease:

Death of spouse	100
Divorce	73
Marital separation	65
Jail term	63
Death of close family member	63
Personal injury or illness	53
Marriage	50
Fired from work	47
Marital reconciliation	45
Retirement	45
Change in family member's health	44
Pregnancy	40
Sex difficulties	39
Addition to family	39
Business readjustment	39
Change in financial status	38
Death of close friend	37
Change to different line of work	36
Change in number of marital arguments	35
Mortgage or loan over $10,000	31
Foreclosure of mortgage or loan	30
Change in work responsibilities	29
Son or daughter leaving home	29
Trouble with in-laws	29
Outstanding personal achievement	28
Spouse begins or stops work	26

Starting or finishing school	26
Change in living conditions	25
Revision of personal habits	24
Trouble with boss	24
Change in work hours, conditions	20
Change in residence	20
Change in schools	20
Change in church activities	19
Change in social activities	18
Mortgage or loan under $10,000	17
Change in sleeping habits	16
Change in number of family gatherings	15
Change in eating habits	15
Vacation	13
Minor violation of law	11

Scoring:

150 or less = 37% chance of getting sick in next 2 years.
150 − 299 = 50% chance of getting ill.
300 + = 80% chance of developing serious illness.

(Adapted from Cheraskin E. Psychodietetics. New York: Stein and Day, 1976.)

Assessment for Nutritional Deficiencies and Excesses

There remains some debate over the actual constitution of optimal nutritional status, as well as the factors that result in it and the tests that can determine it. Nonetheless, it is recognized that a complete biochemical nutrition profile—obtained through the examination of plasma, red blood cells, white blood cells, urine, or tissue—is one of the major components of a comprehensive nutritional assessment.

To augment this examination, it is important to ask the patient a variety of questions regarding the intake of vitamins, minerals, and toxic metals. Questions to help determine the patient's usage pattern and beliefs include:

Do you now use any vitamin or mineral supplements?
Have you ever used any vitamin or mineral supplements?
When and for how long?
What was the dosage and frequency?
Were you consistent in your use?
Why did you take them?
Did they help you?
Are you willing to change your supplement usage?

Common Causes of Nutritional Deficiencies and Excesses

A number of problems and diseases have been linked to the use of vitamins, minerals, and toxic metals. The following is a breakdown of the various deficiencies and excesses associated with each.

Vitamin A deficiency often is associated with:

Protein-calorie malnutrition
Low-fat diet
Steatorrhea (sprue)

Fibrocystic disease of the pancreas
Other pancreatic diseases
Intestinal lipodystrophy (Whipple's disease)
Gluten-induced enteropathy
Intestinal defects after surgery
Cirrhosis of the liver
Infectious diseases—especially when kwashiorkor or marasmus is present
Tuberculosis
Respiratory infections
Pneumonia
Chronic nephritis
Urinary tract infections
Prostatic diseases
Cancer
Diabetes
Myxedema
Night blindness
Xerosis of the conjunctiva
Epithelial keratinization
Corneal dryness
Keratomalacia
Bitot's spots
Impaired hearing
Xerophthalmia
Thickened bone
Loss of lung elasticity
Urinary calculi

Vitamin A excess often is associated with:

Muscle stiffness
Bone tenderness
Precocious skeletal growth
Drowsiness, irritability, fatigue
Headache with increased cerebrospinal fluid pressure
Extensive peeling of the skin
Dry skin
Hair loss
Gingivitis
Vomiting
Anorexia
Enlarged liver
Nystagmus
Hepatosplenomegaly
Enlarged lymph nodes
Slow clotting time
In infants:
   Anorexia
   Irritability
   Dry, itching skin
   Coarse, sparse hair
   Swelling over the long bones
   Enlarged liver

Thiamine (vitamin B₁) deficiency often is associated with:

Chronic alcoholism
Anorexia
Central nervous system changes
Wernicke's encephalopathy
Korsakoff's syndrome
Polyneuritis
Dry beriberi
Wet beriberi
Mental disturbances:
  Irritability
  Nervousness
Muscle weakness
Paralysis of eye muscles
Ataxic gait
Photophobia
Failing vision
Nystagmus
Papilledema
Hemorrhages of retina
Memory defects
Cardiac disturbances
Heart enlargement
Vomiting, diarrhea
Infantile beriberi

Riboflavin (vitamin B₂) deficiency often is associated with:

Alcoholism
Periods of psychological stress
Periods of increased metabolic needs:
  Childhood
  Pregnancy
  Lactation
Pathological stress
Burns
Surgical procedures
Other traumas
Chronic debilitating disease
Congestive heart failure
Hyperthyroidism
Malignancy
Lesion of lip (cheilosis)
Angular stomatitis
Seborrheic dermatitis
Glossitis
Magenta or red tongue
Superficial vascularization of cornea

Niacin, niacinamide (vitamin B₃) deficiency often associated with:

Pellagra
Dermatitis
Diarrhea

Inflammation of mucous membranes
Lassitude
Weakness
Loss of memory
Loss of appetite
Heartburn and other mild digestive disturbances
Slight atrophy or hypertrophy of the papillae
Painful chewing or swallowing
Secondary infection with fuingi or Vincent's organism
Achlorhydria
Profound weight loss
Urethritis with burning, pain, and frequency of urination
Pigmentation
Retarded growth
In females:
  Severe vaginitis
  Amenorrhea
Neurological abnormalities:
  Lack of coordination
  Tremors
  Ataxia
  Reflex disturbances
  Sensory changes
Psychological disturbances:
  Anxiety
  Irritability
  Depression
  Confusion
  Disorientation
  Fearfulness
  Manic/depressive syndrome
  Apathy
  Stupor
  Hyperactivity
  Delusions
  Hallucinations

Niacin, niacinamide (vitamin B$_3$) toxicity often associated with:

Flushing
Dizziness
Nausea

Pantothenic acid deficiency often is associated with:

Psychological disturbances:
  Fatigue
  Irritability
  Restlessness
  Sleep disturbances
  Inability to deal with stress
  Depression
Neurological disturbances:
  Weakness
  Numbness

Neuromotor disturbances
Bilateral paresthesias affecting feet and lower legs and severe pain aggravated by exertion and warmth and alleviated by cold
Muscle cramps
Burning feet
Staggered gait
Gastrointestinal disturbances:
Tachycardia
Cardiovascular instability
Lability of blood pressure with tendency to orthostatic hypotension
Malfunction of stress mechanism
Adrenal cortical hypofunction

Pyridoxine (vitamin B₆) deficiency often is associated with:

Chronic alcoholism
Deficiency as a result of:
Steroid hormones
Oral contraceptives
Hyperthyroidism
Seborrheic dermatitis of eyes, nasolabial folds, mouth
Lesions in face, forehead, skin, behind the ears, scrotal and perineal regions
Intertrigo under breast and other moist areas
Occasionally cheilosis, glossitis, and angular stomatitis
Peripheral neuritis
Psychological disturbances:
Irritability
Depression
Atherosclerosis
Anemia
Infants:
Convulsive seizures
Hyperactivity
Diarrhea

Cobalamin (vitamin B₁₂) deficiency often is associated with:

Pernicious anemia due to lack of the intrinsic factor of Castle in the gastric juice
Malabsorption syndromes:
Sprue
Gluten-induced enteropathy
Intestinal inflammation
Strictures
Anastomoses
Macrocytic anemia
Megaloblastosis of bone marrow
Poor growth
Glossitis
Leukopenia
Neurological abnormalities:
Subacute combined degeneration of spinal cord and peripheral neuritis
Paresthesias involving hands and feet
Degeneration of posterior and lateral columns of spinal cord
Lack of coordination in legs

Loss of fine coordination of fingers
Spastic and either increased or decreased deep tendon reflexes
Sphincter disturbances
Psychological disturbances:
    Irritability
    Memory disturbances
    Depression
    Lessened sense of position and vibration
Tongue—bright red, smooth, sore
Papillae—atrophic
Severe weakness
Severe fatigue
Skin—lemon yellow
Cerebral anoxemia
Cardiovascular complaints:
    Dyspnea
    Chest pain
    Slight edema
    Chronic congestive heart failure
Gastrointestinal symptoms:
    Anorexia
    Nausea
    Vomiting
    Indigestion
    Midepigastric pain
    Diarrhea
    Weight loss occurs occasionally
    Splenomegaly
    Thrombocytopenia

Folic acid, folacin deficiency often is associated with:

Nutritional macrocytic anemia in:
    Pregnancy
    Infancy
    Sprue
    Malabsorption syndromes
Chronic alcoholism
Certain inborn errors of metabolism
Central nervous system changes
Hemoglobinopathies including sickle cell disease, thalassemia (major and
    minor traits)
Intestinal disturbances
Diarrhea
Glossitis
Weight loss
Anorexia in chronic diseases
Syncopal attacks
Leukopenia
Severe pallor of skin
Congestive heart failure with cardiac enlargement
Hepatomegaly
Hyperpigmentation
Thrombocytopenia

Biotin deficiency often is associated with:

Anorexia
Anemia
Dermatitis in scalp, cheeks, neck, groin, gluteal regions
Grayish pallor of skin
Nonpruritic dermatitis
Alopecia in the eye region
Loss of appetite
Hyperesthesia
Nausea
Lassitude
Depression
Muscle pain
Hypercholesterolemia

Choline deficiency often is associated with:

Poor growth
Edema
Impaired cardiovascular system
Memory defects

Inositol deficiency often is associated with:

Alopecia
Failure of growth and lactation
Exudative diathesis
"Spectacled eye" condition

Ascorbic acid (vitamin C) deficiency often is associated with:

Scurvy
In infants (rarely in breast-fed infants; see Chapter 6 for further information):
    Poor appetite
    Irritability
    Bleeding of gums
    Pseudoparalysis
Weakness
Lassitude
Irritability
Aching of joints and muscles
Scorbutic bone formation
Perifollicular hyperkeratotic papules on buttock, thighs, arms, and back
Petechiae
Interruption of lamina dura shown on x-rays of teeth
Hemorrhages of skin, muscles, gums
Edema
Ulcerations of legs
Wounds—lack of healing
Scars—break down
Swollen joints—limited motion
Mucous membranes of gastrointestinal, genitourinary, or respiratory tract tend to bleed
Gums—swollen, red, spongy, ulcerations, bleed easily

Teeth—loosening
Macrocytic anemia with megaloblastosis of bone marrow
Inability to deal with stress
Susceptibility to infections
Depression of immune system
Chronic alcoholism
Chronic diarrhea
Diarrheal diseases

Ascorbic acid (vitamin C) toxicity often is associated with:

Possibly increased risk of renal stones
Possible destruction of vitamin B_{12}
Possible kidney stones in gout patients

Bioflavonoids deficiency often is associated with:

Varicose veins
Capillary fragility

Vitamin D deficiency often is associated with:

In infants (see Chapter 6 for further information):
    Tetany
    Convulsions
    Rickets
    Craniotabes
Osteomalacia
Osteoporosis
Osteodystrophy
Bones—painful, especially lower part of back and legs
Pseudofractures can occur at sites of muscle attachments
Cystlike zones of demineralization in the metaphysical region
Muscular weakness
Bones sensitive to light pressure
Waddling gait
Deformities of pelvis and sacrum
Extensive decalcification
Delayed dentition
Increased alkaline phosphatase

Vitamin D toxicity often is associated with:

Hypercalcemia
Hypercalciuria
Renal calcinosis
Polyuria
Polydipsia
Anorexia
Nausea
Vomiting
Constipation
Thirst
Fatigue
Hypertension
Decreased magnesium

Increased cholesterol
Abnormal electrocardiogram, shortened QT interval
Metastatic calcification

Vitamin E deficiency often is associated with:

Cystic fibrosis of pancreas or congenital atresia of bile ducts
Malabsorption syndromes
Increased creatinuria
Increased hemolysis of red blood cells
Decreased serum lipid levels
Steatorrhea
Xanthomatosis
Biliary cirrhosis
Heart diesease—atherosclerosis
Poor circulation
Muscle weakness
Malnutrition
Infants:
    Anemia
    Decreased levels of tocopherol
    Edema of legs, labia, scrotum

Vitamin E toxicity often is associated with:

Increased action of warfarin
Possible high blood pressure
Increased phosphorus

Vitamin K deficiency often is associated with:

Malabsorption syndromes
Small bowel disease
Steatorrhea
Sprue
Gluten-induced enteropathy
Lesions of small intestine
Short circuiting operations
Chronic pancreatic disease
Hemorrhage
Bleeding from:
    Gums
    Nose
    Gastrointestinal tract
Epistaxis
Ecchymosis
Cutaneous purpura
Prolonged clotting time
Prolonged administration of antibiotics or sulfonamides

Iron deficiency often is associated with:

Listlessness, fatigue, lack of attentiveness
Low performance scores in children
Palpitation on exertion
Decreased work capacity

Sore tongue, angular stomatitis
Koilonychia (thin, concave nails)
Anorexia
Depressed growth
Lowered resistance to infections
Irritability
Geophagia (clay eating)
Hypochromic, microcytic anemia
Normoblastic, hyperplastic bone marrow
Achlorhydria and associated lesions of the gastrointestinal tract
Degenerative changes in stomach parietal cells
Menorrhagia
Increased incidence of respiratory infections
Cardiac hypertrophy with copper deficiency

Iron excess is associated with:

Fibrosis
Skin pigmentation
Ascorbic acid depletion
Severe siderosis plus scurvy can cause osteoporosis

Copper deficiency often is associated with:

Hypochromic, microcytic anemia
Decreased growth
Protein deficiency
Kwashiorkor
Cardiac diseases
Cardiovascular lesions
Atherosclerosis
Aortic rupture due to improper elastin formation
Cirrhosis and associated cholangeitis
Infectious hepatitis
Dermatosis
Decreased melanin production leading to loss of hair color, albinism, baldness
Osteoporosis, fractures, bone deformities
Hypothyroid function
Decreased fertility
Pancreatic lesions
GI disturbances
Long-term parenteral hyperalimentation can deplete copper
Excessive urinary or fecal losses

Copper excess is associated with:

Aplastic enemia
Thalassemia
Nephritis
Wilson's disease
Various types of liver diseases
Schizophrenia
Eczema
Rheumatoid arthritis
Toxicosis of pregnancy
Sickle cell anemia

Zinc deficiency often is associated with:

Retarded growth
Delayed wound healing
Severe thermal burns
Eczema, skin rashes
Parakeratosis
Alopecia
Delayed onset of puberty and sexual development
Decreased milk production during lactation
Weak labor
Mental retardation
Emotional disturbances
Decreased learning ability
Anorexia
Hypogeusia
Diarrhea
Stress of disease or trauma may adversely affect a marginal zinc deficiency
Repeated infections
Cirrhosis
Chronic leukemia
Multiple myeloma
Pernicious anemia
Psoriasis
Venous leg ulceration
Atherosclerosis
Malignant tumors
Myocardial infarction
Pneumonia
Active tuberculosis
Chronic sepsis
Decubitus ulcers
Uremia
Malabsorption
Dwarfism
Raynaud's disease
Arthritis
Hypertension
Diabetes
Birth defects (skeletal)

Zinc excess is associated with:

Problems in mineralization of bone growth
Growth depression

Chromium deficiency may be associated with:

Decreased weight gain
Atherosclerosis
Disturbed lipid metabolism
Protein-calorie malnutrition
Increased serum cholesterol
Increased incidence of aortic plaques
Impaired glucose tolerance
Corneal lesions

Selenium deficiency has been associated with:

Retarded growth
Kwashiorkor
Infections
Infertility in animals
Increased plasma cholesterol
Necrotic changes in liver
Increased severity of cataracts

Selenium toxicity is associated with:

Discolored and decayed teeth
Yellow skin color
Chronic arthritis
Edema
Lassitude
Garlic odor on breath
Liver or renal damage
Skin eruptions
Atrophic brittle nails

Manganese deficiency may be associated with:

Bone disorders
Diabetes
Rheumatoid arthritis
Rickets
Jaundice
Ataxia, poor equilibrium
Dizziness
Atherosclerotic lesions
Reproduction dysfunctions
Lowered defensive responses
Retarded skeletal growth
Increased fat deposition
Increased blood cholesterol

Manganese excess is associated with (usually found only with contaminated well water):

Decreased appetite
Neurological disorders
Psychological disorders

Calcium deficiency may be associated with:

Rickets
Scleroderma
Eczema
Brittle fingernails
Acromegaly
Poor blood coagulation
Poor appetite
Intestinal stasis
Hyperhydrosis

Hypocalcemic tetany
Aching joint pain
Osteomalacia and fractures
Impairments of spinal column
Tooth decay, periodontal disease
Hypertension
Myocardosis
Increased flouride retention
Increased lead retention
Hay fever, asthma
Increased parathyroid activity
Rheumatoid arthritis
Increased blood cholesterol, triglycerides, phospholipids
Increased blood pressure and body temperature

Hypercalcemia is associated with:

Primary hyperthyroidism
Vitamin D toxicity
Sarcoidosis
Adrenal failure
Graves' disease
Malignant tumors
Burnett's syndrome
Bone metastases
Artificial menopause

Magnesium deficiency is associated with:

Alcoholism
Malabsorption syndromes
Diuretic therapy
Loss of potassium
Pregnancy
Atherosclerosis
Thrombosis
Viral hepatitis
Chronic myelogenous leukemia
Protein-calorie malnutrition
Postsurgical or burn patients
Diabetic acidosis and coma
Hypertension
Hypercholesterolemia
Congestive heart failure
Cardiac arrhythemia
Cirrhosis
Tetany
Addison's disease
Epilepsy
Oral contraceptive use
Metastatic calcification
Malignant tumors
Hyperparathyroidism
Eclampsia
Intestinal malabsorption

Neuromuscular excitability
Depression
Renal insufficiency (acute nephritis and renal amyloidosis)
Lowered appetite
Insomnia
Hypercalcemia
Muscle tremors, twitching
Cardiovascular changes
Increased serum cholesterol
Reduced growth
Hyperirritability
Personality changes and emotional crises
Skin lesions
Potassium depletion
Confusion, disorientation
Bone weakening in the elderly
Decrease in blood pressure and body temperature

Magnesium excess is associated with:

Renal diseases
Adrenal insufficiency
Uremia
Jaundice
Depression of nervous system
Mental retardation
Antecedent gastroenteritis

Sodium depletion may be associated with:

Reproductive disorders
Decrease in basal metabolism
Decreased growth
Dermatosis
Eye disturbances
Anorexia
Weakness, lassitude
Increased blood urea
Hypotension
Severe cardiovascular distress or exertion
Decreased extracellular fluid volume
Decrease in hydrochloric acid concentration
Increase in adrenocortical activity
Polycythemia
Aberrations of flavor
Loss of weight
Muscular cramps
Decreased resistance to infection

Sodium excess may be associated with:

Increased blood pressure
Shortened life span
Edema
Polydipsia

Weight gain
Renal failure
Atherosclerosis
Distrurbed lipid metabolism
Congestive heart failure
Anorexia
Increased evidence of hypertension
Decrease in adrenergic activity
Diabetics with severe acidosis
Bronchial asthma

Potassium may be depleted after:

Use of diuretics
Diabetes mellitus
Cancer
Renal loss
Inadequate dietary intake
Use of highly processed foods
Magnesium deficiency
Diarrhea, loss of fluid from the gastrointestinal tract

Potassium depletion is associated with:

Hypokalemia
Alkalosis
Muscular dystrophy
Renal and cardiac lesions
Arthritis
Retarded growth
Edema, salt retention
Muscle weakness, paralysis
Decreased protein synthesis
Degeneration of mesenchyme tissue
Increased cholesterol levels
Respiratory distress (pulmonary disease, bronchial asthma)
Decreased blood pressure, cardiac output, stroke volume, renal blood flow

Lead

Acute exposure to high amounts can result in toxicity

Symptoms of lead toxicity or poisoning include:

Severe tremors
Vertigo
Motor palsy
Optic neuritis
General mental disturbances

If untreated it may result in:

Ataxia
Convulsions
Death
In children:

Vomiting
Drowsiness
Stupor
Hyperirritability
Anorexia
General mental disturbances
Recurrent seizures
Cerebral palsy
Learning difficulties

Lead

Signs and symptoms of subclinical poisoning include:

In children:
Hyperactivity
Temper tantrums
Fearfulness
Listlessness
Emotional and behavioral problems
In adults:
Anorexia
Muscle discomfort
Headache
Constipation or diarrhea
Insomnia
Abdominal pains

Mercury

Signs and symptoms of toxicity include:

Gingivitis
Stomatitis
Metallic taste in mouth
Loss of appetite
Progressive renal damage
Hypertension
Behavioral changes
Depression
Irritability
Insomnia
Fatigue

Cadmium

Signs and symptoms of toxicity include:

Decreased appetite
Mouth lesions
Loss of hair
Lung damage
Dry, scaling skin
Hypertension
Decreased body temperature
Decreased growth

Decreased milk production in lactation
Decreased testosterone activity
Anemia, proteinuria, glucosuria
Anosmia

Arsenic

Signs and symptoms of toxicity include:

Weakness
Diarrhea
Anorexia
Skin pigmentation
Edema
Dermatitis
Numbness
Keratosis of palms and soles
Inhibited wound healing
Garlic odor on breath
Peripheral neuritis
Severe thirst
Difficulty in swallowing

Assessment for Physical Abnormalities

The comprehensive nutritional analysis continues with a complete physical examination. In this clinical portion of the evaluation, the examining doctor should pay special attention to those areas that regularly display signs of poor nutritional status: the skin, eyes, lips, mouth, gums, tongue, hair, and nails. Other points of particular interest to the practitioner include the patient's height, weight, blood pressure, glands, subcutaneous tissue, musculoskeletal system, gastrointestinal system, nervous system, and cardiovascular system.

Aspects to be evaluated during a total examination include the following:

Is the skin smooth, slightly moist, and of good color? Is it pale, dry, scaly, and hyperpigmented? Is there evidence of rashes, pellagrous dermatitis, or decubiti? Are there any dark or light spots? Does the patient have dry or pale mucous membranes or decreased skin turgor?

Are the eyes bright and clear, with pink conjunctiva? Are they sunken, dull, and dry? Is there evidence of blindness or night blindness? Are there any prominant blood vessels or mound of tissue or sclera?

Are the lips moist and of good color? Are they cracked, chapped, dry, swollen, or red? Is there evidence of fissures or bleeding?

Are the gums pink and firm? Are they red, sore, spongy, swollen, or receding? Do they bleed easily?

Is the tongue pink with papillae present? Is it smooth, slick, raw, purple, magenta, or white? Does it have a gray coating? Is it beefy red or fissured?

Is the hair normally distributed, firmly attached, shiny, and lustrous? Is it dry, thin, or dull? Is it depigmented? Can it be easily plucked without pain? Does the patient describe hair changes?

Are the nails firm and pink? Are they spoon shaped (koilonychia), brittle, or ridged? Does the patient say they have changed?

Are there normal amounts of fat in the subcutaneous tissue? Is there evidence of edema?

Is there any evidence of growth retardation? Is the weight ideal or normal for the patient's age?

Have the patient's muscles and bones developed normally? Is there good muscle tone? Complaints of calf muscle tenderness or weak thighs? Any sign of muscle wasting, twitching, pain, or cramps? Evidence of fractures, osteoporosis, or paralysis?

Are there any palpable organs or masses (except in children, where the liver edge may be palpable)? Is there evidence of hepatosplenomegaly? Does the patient experience difficulty chewing or swallowing?

Are either the face, cheeks, or front of neck swollen?

Are the patient's reflexes normal? Is there motor weakness, or loss of vibration or position sense? Has the patient described burning or tingling in the hands or feet?

Are the patient's heart rate and rhythm normal? Are there murmurs? Any evidence of cardiac enlargement, tachycardia, cardiomegaly, or congestive heart failure?

Is blood pressure normal for the patient's age?

Once these questions have been answered, the examining doctor can correlate results with the corresponding nutritional problem. Remember, however, that such clinical signs may be mild and nonspecific, or they may stem from a variety of nutritional deficiencies. In addition, some of these physical abnormalities also may be the consequence of nonnutritional factors.

Skin-Face

Seborrhea, nasolabial—Scaling of skin with dry, gray, yellow, or greasy material around the nostrils. Consider deficiency of niacin, pyridoxine, ribloflavin.

Follicular hyperkeratosis—Blocked follicles with plugs of keratin. Consider deficiency of vitamins A and C or of essential fatty acids.

Erythematous eruption—Sunburnlike condition of skin. Consider excess of vitamin A.

Diffuse depigmentation—A lightening of the skin color, especially on the center of the face. Consider protein-calorie malnutrition.

Moon face—Mouth looks "pursed in" due to rounded prominence of cheeks. Consider protein-calorie malnutrition associated with kwashiorkor in children.

Skin-General

Dry, scaling skin—Consider deficiency of vitamin A, zinc, essential fatty acids. Consider excess of vitamin A.

Hyperpigmentation—Color of skin changes to red and then to brown. Consider pellagra, niacin deficiency, and protein-calorie malnutrition associated with kwashiorkor.

Follicular hyperkeratosis—Follicles become blocked with plugs of keratin derived from their epithelial lining that has undergone squamous metaplasia. Consider deficiencies of vitamins A and C or of essential fatty acids.

Flaky paint dermatosis—Skin becomes hyperpigmented and keratin separates in flakes. Consider protein-calorie malnutrition.

Petechiae, purpura—Small, pinhead-sized hemorrhages in the skin that are characterized by red spots which then turn purple. Consider deficiencies of vitamins C and K.

Yellow pigmentation sparing sclerae (benign)—Yellow color in skin especially seen on palms of hands. Consider carotene or vitamin A excess.

Pellagrous dermatosis—Red swollen pigmentation of areas exposed to sunlight. Consider nicotinic acid deficiency.

Edema—Seen in protein-energy malnutrition with hypoalbuminemia and in wet beriberi due to thiamine deficiency. Also consider deficiencies of protein and Vitamin E (in premature infants).

Excessive bruising—Due to increased fragility of capillary walls. Consider vitamin K deficiency.

Poor wound healing—Consider deficiencies of protein-energy, zinc, possible essential fatty acids, riboflavin (scrotal and vulval), pyridoxine (nasolabial).

Poor tissue turgor—Consider water deficiency.

Thickening of skin—Consider essential fatty acid deficiency.

Eyes

Bitot's spots—Grayish or glistening white plaques formed from desquamated thickened conjunctival epithelium. Usually bilateral, more common in children. Consider vitamin A deficiency.

Pale conjunctiva—Eyelids, whites of eyes and inner surface of cheeks become pale. Symptoms of anemia. Consider iron, folic acid, or vitamin B_{12} deficiency.

Conjunctival xerosis—The whites of the eye and inner lids become dry, rough, and pigmented. Eye appears wrinkled when rotated. Associated with vitamin A deficiency.

Corneal xerosis—The conjunctiva of the eye is dry, opaque, and translucent. Consider vitamin A deficiency.

Keratomalacia—Softening of the cornea. Eye becomes opaque. Nightblindness. Consider vitamin A deficiency.

Angular palpebritis—Inflammation of eyelids. Corners of eye become red, cracked. Often correlated with angular stomatitis. Consider deficiency of riboflavin, niacin.

Band keratitis—Whitish or grayish band extending across the cornea. Consider an increase in serum calcium and an excess of vitamin D.

Scleral icterus, mild—Jaundice of the white or sclerotic outer coat of the eye. Consider deficiency of pyridoxine.

Papilledema—Edema and inflammation of the optic nerve at its point of entrance into the eyeball. Consider excess of vitamin A.

Corneal arcus—White ring around the eye. Consider deficiency of hyperlipidemia.

Corneal vascularization—Consider riboflavin deficiency.

Xanthelasma—Small yellowish lumps around the eyes. Consider deficiency of hyperlipidemia.

Blepharitis—Consider B-complex deficiency.

Ophthalmoplegia—Consider thiamine deficiency.

Photophobia—Consider zinc deficiency.

Lips, Mouth, Gums

Angular stomatitis—Redness, cracking and flaking at the corners of the mouth. Significant if bilateral only. Rule out poor dentures, syphilis, herpes. Consider riboflavin, niacin, pyridoxine, and iron deficiency.

Angular scars—Pink or white scars at corners of mouth resulting from healed lesions. Consider riboflavin, protein, B-complex, or iron deficiency.

Cheilosis—Vertical cracks in center of lip. Lips are swollen and buccal mucosa seems to extend out onto the lip, which also may be ulcerated. Consider deficiency of riboflavin, thiamine.

Ulcers of mouth—An open lesion of the mouth. Consider vitamin C deficiency.

Scorbutic gums—Gums are red, spongy, with possible bleeding. Rule out chronic overdoses of hydantoinates (Dilantin, etc.), poor hygiene, and lymphoma. Consider vitamin C deficiency.

Spongy, bleeding, receding gums—Consider vitamin C deficiency.

Tongue

Papillary atrophy—Tongue is smooth, pale, slick. Taste buds atrophied. Rule out nonnutritional anemia. Consider deficiency of folate, riboflavin, iron, vitamin B_{12}.

Magenta tongue—Tongue becomes beefy, purplish red. Consider deficiency of riboflavin.

Scarlet or raw tongue—Consider deficiency of nicotinic acid.

Fissures—Cracks on tongue surface, lack of taste buds on sides or bottom of cracks. Indicates a definite break in epithelium. Consider niacin deficiency.

Glossitis—Tongue is beefy, red, painful. Taste buds are atrophied. Taste changes include hypersensitivity and burning, especially when eating. Consider deficiency of niacin, folic acid, riboflavin, iron, vitamin B_{12}, pyridoxine, and tryptophan.

Swollen or large-size tongue—Consider deficiency of niacin, iodine.

Hair

Thin, fine, sparse—Consider deficiency of protein, biotin, zinc. Consider excess of vitamin A.

Easy pluckability—A clump of hair may be pulled out easily and with no pain. Consider protein deficiency.

Lackluster—Dull, dry, brittle. Consider vitamin A deficiency.

Flag sign, traverse depigmentation—Lightening of hair in alternating bands. Consider deficiency of protein, copper.

Coiled, corkscrewlike—Consider deficiency of vitamins A and C.

Nails

White spots—Random spots of white on nails. Consider zinc deficiency.

Brittle nails—Nails are hard and break easily. Consider protein-calorie malnutrition.

Koilonychia—Nails become shaped like spoons. Rule out Plummer-Vinson syndrome and clubbing from cardiopulmonary disease. Consider iron deficiency.

Ridging—Nails have ridges. Consider calcium deficiency, deficiency of HCL.

Subcutaneous Tissue

Amount of subcutaneous tissue—This can be measured with skinfold calipers. Excess fat creates prominent body folds where friction between skin surfaces and maceration from accumulated moisture leads to intertrigo. Infection of these areas by *Staphylococci*, *Candida* and superficial dermatophytes is common in obese, diabetic patients. In the obese the thickened subcutaneous fat layer makes heat dissipation more difficult and sweating is increased. Miliaria rubra and other sweat retention problems are found more often in the obese.

Edema—Swelling, usually of ankles and feet (bilaterally). If the tissues are pressed on for 3 seconds, edematous tissue will pit. Consider sodium and water retention, pregnancy, protein deficiency, vitamin B_6 deficiency, protein losing enteropathy, varicose veins, and thiamine deficiency.

Malnutrition associated with starvation, anorexia nervosa, or prolonged wasting—Skin becomes pale, thin, loose, inelastic. Cool to touch, tendency to cyanosis in cold weather. Dryness accompanied by scaling and fine mosaic fissuring. Occasionally follicular hyperkeratosis. Abnormalities of pigmentation may be seen as hypermelanosis with predominance of high-exposed areas.

Height, Weight

Growth retardation—Consider deficiencies of protein-energy, magnesium, zinc, vitamin D, calcium.

Anorexia—Consider deficiencies of vitamins B_{12} and C, chloride, sodium, thiamine.

Fat above standard—Consider obesity.

Fat below standard—Consider starvation, marasmus.

Muscular and Skeletal Systems

Frontal and parietal bossing—Round swelling or thickening of head in infants. Head becomes larger than normal. Consider previous vitamin D deficiency.

Beading of ribs—Enlargement of costochondral junctions of the ribs produces what is termed "rachitic rosary." Small lumps can be seen on chest wall. Consider active deficiency of vitamin D and calcium.

Knock-knees or bowed legs—Legs are either curved outward at knees or bowed inward. Rule out congenital deformities. Consider previous deficiency of vitamin D, calcium.

Epiphyseal enlargement—Ends of long bones enlarge at wrist, ankles, and knees. Rule out renal disease, malabsorption, trauma, congenital deficiency; consider active vitamin D deficiency. If painful, consider vitamin C deficiency.

Muscle wasting—Body skeleton prominent. Can be measured by upper arm measurements. Consider protein-calorie malnutrition.

Craniotabes—Seen in children under 1 year of age. Softening of skull in occipital and parietal bones along the lambdoidal sutures. Consider active vitamin D deficiency.

Persistently open anterior fontanelle—A soft spot on baby's head that does not harden by 18 months. Rule out hydrocephalus. Consider active vitamin D deficiency.

Diffuse skeletal deformities—Pain in bones, particularly in lower part of back and legs. Bones soft, tender due to failure of mineralization. Consider osteomalacia, vitamin D deficiency.

Deformities of the thorax—Pigeon chest and Harrison's sulcus (a horizontal depression along the lower border of the chest). Consider previous vitamin D deficiency.

Harrison's groove—Retraction of the rib cage at the attachment of the diaphragm. Rule out chronic respiratory infection. Consider Vitamin D deficiency.

Musculoskeletal hemorrhages—Bleeding into the muscles. Check by further testing. Consider vitamin C deficiency.

Calf muscle tenderness, weak thighs—Consider thiamine deficiency.

Muscular twitching—Consider pyridoxine deficiency.

Muscular pains—Consider deficiencies of biotin, selenium.

Muscular weakness—Consider deficiencies of sodium, potassium.

Muscular cramps—Consider deficiencies of sodium, chloride.

Gastrointestinal System

Bloated stomach—Associated with deficiency of pancreatic enzymes, HCL, food allergies.

Hepatomegaly—Enlarged liver. Prevalent in many conditions. Consider chronic malnutrition with protein deficiency.

Glands

Parotid enlargement—Gland just below earlobe. Chronic enlargement. Significant if bilateral. Consider protein deficiency.

Thyroid—May be visible when patient's head is tipped backward. Rule out cysts, tumors, and hyperthyroidism. Consider iodine deficiency.

Adrenal glands—Adrenal insufficiency is manifested by weight loss, weakness, loss of body hair in the female, reactive hypoglycemia after ohydrate meal, and occasionally hypercalcemia.

Pancreas—A racemose compound gland that secretes insulin and pancreatic juices. Insulin is one of the hormones that controls the metabolism of carbohydrates. Hyperfunction of the islands of Langerhans can result in hypoglycemia whereas hypofunction will result in diabetes mellitus.

Nervous System

Irritability—Often for no reason, patient reacts strongly to minor events. Consider deficiency of vitamins B_1, B_3, potassium, magnesium, calcium; hypoglycemia, food allergies.

Depression—Consider deficiency of vitamins B_1, B_2, B_3, pantothenic acid.

Inability to concentrate—Consider deficiency of vitamins B_1, B_{12}, protein.

Memory loss—Consider deficiency of choline, inositol, lecithin and vitamin B_6.

Insomnia—Consider deficiency of vitamins B_3, B_6, C, folic acid; hypoglycemia; food allergies.

Sensory loss and motor weakness—Consider deficiency of vitamin B_1, potassium, calcium, magnesium and manganese.

Loss of vibratory sense—Rule out peripheral neuropathy due to other causes. Consider deficiency of vitamins B_1, B_{12}.

Loss of knee use and reflexes—Rule out peripheral neuropathy due to other causes. Consider deficiency of vitamins B_1, B_{12}.

Burning and tingling of hands and feet—Consider thiamine deficiency.

Cardiovascular System

Tachycardia—Rapid heart beat (over 100). Consider food allergies, thiamine deficiency (wet beriberi), anemia. Consider deficiency of calcium, potassium, magnesium.

Cardiac enlargement—Enlarged heart, usually non-nutritional. May occur in anemia and wet beriberi.

Decreased cardiac function—Consider phosphorous deficiency.

Elevated blood pressure—Consider sodium intake.

Suggested Readings

Abboud IA, Osman HG. Vitamin A and xerosis. Exp Eye Res 1968;7:388–393.

Anonymous. Nutritional assessment: what is it, how is it used? (Report) The Ross Medical Nutritional System, Ross Laboratories, October 1987.

Austin JE. The perilous journey of nutritional evaluation. Am J Clin Nutr 1978;72(5):497–501.

Barrocas A, Bain GE. Human biotin deficiency induced by raw egg consumption in a cirrhotic patient. Am J Clin Nutr 1968;21:173.

Beal VA. Nutrition in the life span. New York: John Wiley and Sons, 1980.

Bean WB, Hodges RE. Pantothenic acid deficiency induced in human subjects. J Clin Invest 1955;34:1073–1084.

Bennion M. Clinical nutrition. New York: Harper & Row, 1979.

Binder HJ, Spiro HM. Tocopherol deficiency in man. Am J Clin Nutr 1967;20:594–601.

Blackburn GL, Bothe A. Nutritional assessment and patient outcome during oncological therapy. Cancer (Phila) 1979;43:2065–2069.

Butterworth CE. The dimensions of clinical nutrition. Am J Clin Nutr 1975;28:943.

Christakis G. Nutritional assessment in health programs. Washington: American Public Health Association Inc., 1974.

Cole M, Turner A. Extraocular palsy and thiamine therapy in Wernicke's encephalopathy. Am J Clin Nutr 1969;22:44–51.

Comaish S. Metabolic disorders and hair growth. Br J Dermatol 1971;84:83–86.

Committee on Nutrition, American Academy of Pediatrics. Prophylactic requirement and the toxicity of vitamin D. Pediatrics 1963;31:512–525.

Coursin DB. Present status of vitamin B_6 metabolism. Am J Clin Nutr 1961;9:304.

Davidson S, Passmore R. Human nutrition and dietetics. New York: Churchill Livingstone, 1975.

DeLuca HF, Schnoes HK. Metabolism and mechanism of action of vitamin D. Ann Rev Biochem 1976;45:631–666.

DeLuca HF, Suttie JW, eds. The fat soluable vitamins. Madison, Wisconsin: University of Wisconsin Press, 1969.

Department of Health, Education and Welfare. April 1975. Preliminary findings of the first Health and Nutritional Examination Survey, USA, 1971–72: Anthropometric and clinical findings. PHS, DHEW Publication No. (HRA) 75–1229.

Dreizen S. Oral indications of the deficiency states. Postgrad Med 1971;49:97–102.

Escott-Stump S. Nutrition and diagnosis-related care. 2nd ed. Philadelphia: Lea & Febiger, 1988.

Foulds WS, Chisholm IA. The optic neuropathy of pernicious anemia. Arch Ophthalmol 1969;82:427–432.

Galante L, Colston KW. The regulation of vitamin D metabolism. Nature (Lond) 1973;244:438–440.

Goldsmith GA. Niacin-tryptophan relationships in man and niacin requirement. Am J Clin Nutr 1958;6:479–486.

Goldsmith GA. Clinical aspects of riboflavin deficiency. In: Rivlin RS, ed. Monograph on riboflavin. New York: Plenum, 1975.

Halpern SL. Quick reference to clinical nutrition. Philadelphia: JB Lippincott, 1979.

Harvey KB, Blumenkrantz MJ. Nutritional assessment and treatment of chronic renal failure. Am J Clin Nutr 1980;33:1586–1597.

Herbert V. Folic acid deficiency: introduction. Am J Clin Nutr 1970;23:841–842.

Hodges RE, Baker EM. Experimental scurvy in man. Am J Clin Nutr 1969;22:535–548.

Hodges RE, Hood J. Clinical manifestations of ascorbic acid deficiency in man. Am J Clin Nutr 1971;24:432–443.

Jelliffe D. The assessment of the nutritional status of the community. World Health Organization monograph, Ser. No. 53, Geneva, 1966.

Kamel W. The nature of vitamin A deficiency in Jordan and Bangladesh. In: Vitamin deficiency and and blindness prevention. American Foundation for the Overseas Blind, May 1974.

Krause MV, Mahan LK. Food, nutrition, and diet therapy: a textbook of nutritional care. 7th ed. Philadelphia: WB Saunders, 1984.

Lerner M, Lerner A. Psoriasis and protein intake. Arch Dermatol 1964;90:217–225.

Logan, WS. Vitamin A and keratinization. Arch Dermatol 1972;105:748–753.

Lowenstein FW. Preliminary clinical and anthropometric findings from the first Health and Nutrition Examination Survey, USA, 1971–72. Am J Clin Nutr 1976;29:918.

McLaren DS. Involvement of the eye in protein malnutrition. Bull WHO 1958;19:303–314.

McLaren DS. Xerophthalmia: a neglected problem. Nutr Rev 1964;22:289–291.

Mistry SP, Dakshinamutri K. Biochemistry of biotin. Vitamins and hormones: advances in research and application 1964;22:1–55.

Muncie HL, Sobal J. The vitamin-mineral supplement history. Fam Prac 1987;4:365–368.

Nagaraju M, Adamson D. Skin manifestation of folic acid deficiency. Br J Dermatol 1971;84:32–36.

Nizel AE. Nutrition and oral problems. World Rev Nutr Diet 1973;16:226–252.

Noguchi T, Cantor AH. Mode of action of selenium and vitamin E in prevention of exudative diathesis in chicks. J Nutr 1973;103:1502–1511.

Norman AW, Haussler TH. Basic studies on the mechanism of action of vitamin D. Am J Clin Nutr 1969;22:396–411.

Olson J. The biological role of vitamin A in maintaining epithelial tissues. Israel J Med Sci 1972;8:1170–1178.

Pauling L. Vitamin C and the common cold. San Francisco: W.H. Freeman and Company, 1970.

Prasad AS. Trace elements in human health and disease, vol I, II. New York: Academic Press, 1976.

Press M, Kikuchi H. Diagnosis and treatment of essential fatty acid deficiency in man. Br Med J 1974;2:247–250.

Reynolds EH, Rothfeld P. Neurological disease associated with folate deficiency. Br Med J 1973;2:398–400.

Roe D. Nutritional significance of generalized exfoliative dermatoses. NY State J Med 1962;62:3455–3457.

Sandstead HH, Carter JP. How to diagnose nutritional disorders in daily practice. Nutr Today 1969;4:20.

Schneider HA, Anderson CE, Corsin DB. Nutritional support of medical practice. Hagerstown, Maryland: Harper and Row, 1977.

Shils ME, Young VR, eds. Modern nutrition in health and disease. 7th ed. Philadelphia: Lea & Febiger, 1988.

Simko MD, Cowell C, Gilbride JA. Nutritional assessment: a comprehensive guide for planning intervention. Rockville, Maryland: Aspen Publishers Inc, 1984.

Stahl SS. Nutritional influences on periodontal disease. World Rev Nutr Diet 1971;13:277.

Tickner A, Basit A. Vitamin C and exfoliative dermatitis. Br J Dermatol 1960;72:403–408.

Underwood EJ. Trace elements in human and animal nutrition, 3rd ed. New York: Academic Press, 1971.

Weinsier RL, Butterworth CE. Handbook of clinical nutrition. St. Louis: CV Mosby, 1981.

2

Evaluation Of Dietary Intake

A comprehensive dietary evaluation is as important as any other aspect of the total nutritional assessment. Such a careful analysis is critical because the patient may have inadequate or less than optimal nutritional status without any overt symptoms. Therefore, describing the situation in general terms (i.e., "the patient is well nourished and well developed" or "the patient seems to have a satisfactory diet") simply is not sufficient.

To gain information that will lead to an accurate assessment of nutritional status, the practitioner must completely evaluate the patient's typical dietary intake. This includes a detailed accounting of all foods, beverages, and additives consumed, as well as an accurate portrayal of all preparation methods and the eating habits that led to their consumption. In addition to its invaluable help in the complicated process of painting a composite portrait of the patient, this procedure also is useful in the reinforcement of any positive nutritional behaviors that already may be practiced.

Creation of a truly accurate evaluation, however, usually is considered to be the most difficult part of any nutritional assessment. It is hard to record the patient's dietary intake without affecting it, for example, because eating habits often change when they are being monitored. Many patients also fail to accurately record all of the food that they consume, either because they forget or because they misunderstand the directions. And a variety of other factors—ranging from cooking methods to food manufacturing processes—can vary greatly from patient to patient and have a severe impact on the end result.

In addition, specific difficulties often begin early in life and continue for a long period of time before clinical symptoms become apparent. But at that time, such difficulties may not even appear related to the illness, or they ultimately may contribute to it without being readily identified as the cause. In any comprehensive nutritional evaluation, therefore, the clinician also must consider the insidious factor of time in combination with the marginal nutritional intake that ultimately can lead to degenerative disease.

Finally, any pattern of craving, eating, bingeing, or starving that is exhibited by the patient also must be fully analyzed. Many patients, for example, exhibit periods of bingeing followed by periods of severe restriction of foods; these episodes often are triggered by excess stress, psychological tension, weight gain, or repressed food allergies. Despite the various obstacles that often stand in the way of the examination of these incidents, the clinician must be able to determine all of the causes and patterns of food intake in order to prevent these negative habits from predominating.

Due to these and related complications, the reliability of any dietary intake evaluation may be suspect. Thus, such evaluations—in and of themselves—rarely provide sufficient information with which to fully determine a patient's nutritional status. In conjunction with other verbal, physical, and laboratory examinations, though, all of the data that is uncovered through them will help to confirm a diagnosis and serve as a starting point for appropriate treatment.

At the present time, there are several different methods that can be used to obtain a dietary history. In turn, this dietary history allows the practitioner to define the problem, uncover areas of deficiency, and develop a nutritional profile for the patient. In determining which form of dietary assessment to employ, the clinician must take into account the following factors:

The degree of accuracy of each method.

The ability of the patient to use the various methods; important factors to consider are the patient's age and level of education, and the amount of food that the patient reports eating in restaurants.

The time needed by the patient to complete each method.

The expense of each method.

Once the appropriate method is selected, data derived from it can be evaluated along with baseline information determined through the case history and physical examination that are detailed in Chapter 1.

Comparison of Dietary Intake Assessment Methods

Method 1: Weighing Method

This method involves duplicate analysis. The patient cooks each meal and divides it in half; one-half is then eaten while the other half is analyzed for amounts of nutrients present.

Advantages	Disadvantages
1. High degree of of accuracy.	1. Complicated method that takes a great deal of time on the part of the patient.
	2. Selectivity on respondents willing to participate.
	3. Elderly, children, and those who eat in restaurants can not cooperate easily.
	4. Very costly.

Method 2: Records of Menus, 7-Day Diary

This method entails the patient's recording of all foods and beverages consumed during a specific period of time, such as 24 hours or 1 week (see Figs. 2.1 and 2.2). The recording should be done immediately after the foods and beverages are consumed. Portion sizes are estimated using food models and standard measuring instruments, or they actually are weighed. When the patient returns to the practitioner's office, this record is then discussed.

Advantages	Disadvantages
1. Low cost.	1. Resistance of patient to maintaining diary.
2. Little time is needed.	
3. Convenient (can record in pocket notebook or on forms).	2. Omissions of certain items such as salad dressings, gravies, etc. are common.
4. Can be used in restaurants.	

24-HOUR FOOD DIARY

Name: _____ Date: _____

DIRECTIONS:
1. Write down everything you ate or drank yesterday from the time you got up until you went to bed. It may help you remember by thinking about the time of day: breakfast, mid-morning, lunch, afternoon, dinner, and before bed.
2. Write down what time and where you ate or drank each food.
3. Describe each food fully. Tell whether it was raw or cooked. If cooked, tell how it was prepared (for example: fried, boiled). Also, tell what it was served with (for example: with cream sauce, with french dressing).
4. For casseroles or mixed dishes, list the major ingredients (for example: Hamburger casserole—hamburger, macaroni, tomatoes, onions).
5. Write down the amount of each food and beverage. Please give the amounts in ounces, tablespoons, or units (e.g. *slice* bread, *1 medium* apple). (Do not give the amount as 1 bowl, 1 glass, etc.). If you are uncertain about the quantity, please estimate.

EXAMPLE

TIME	PLACE	FOOD EATEN	AMOUNT

6:30 p.m.	Home	Toasted Cheese sandwich made with
		  whole wheat bread
		  cheese, American processed
		  margarine
		Cream of Tomato soup—Campbells
		  made with whole milk
		Peanut Butter Cookies
			2 slices
			1 slice
			1 tablespoon
			1 8-ounce bowl
			
			3 (2″ size)

TIME	PLACE	FOOD EATEN	AMOUNT

Wisconsin Div. of Health, WIC program, Revised 3/79
Figure 2.1.   24-Hour food diary. A 1-day food diary, filled out by the patient, will help the practitioner determine dietary patterns and habits.

3. Time consuming for both patient and practitioner.
4. Recording process itself may lead to alterations by patient.
5. If recording period is brief (i.e., 24 hours), it may give a poor estimate of patient's habitual intake.
6. Patients must be literate.

SEVEN DAY FOOD DIARY

Name   Date

Time	Food Eaten—Symptoms	Urine pH	Defecation	Time	Food Eaten—Symptoms	Urine pH	Defecation
12:00 AM				12:00 PM			
1:00 AM				1:00 PM			
2:00 AM				2:00 PM			
3:00 AM				3:00 PM			
4:00 AM				4:00 PM			
5:00 AM				5:00 PM			
6:00 AM				6:00 PM			
7:00 AM				7:00 PM			
8:00 AM				8:00 PM			
9:00 AM				9:00 PM			
10:00 AM				10:00 PM			
11:00 AM				11:00 PM			

Figure 2.2.   7-Day food diary. More complete dietary information can be assessed by means of a full week's food diary, 1 day's example of which is reproduced here.

Method 3: Time Period Recalls

This method utilizes the patient's memory of all foods and beverages consumed during a specific time, such as 24 hours. Methods of preparation and additives that are used also are recalled. Open-ended questions should be asked by the practitioner, and intake can be recorded on a blank piece of paper. This method often is used in large-scale nutritional surveys.

Advantages
1. Very inexpensive.
2. Less time needed by the patient than for dietary records.
3. Better cooperation on the part of the patient.
4. Suitable for use with illiterate patients as well as the aged (except when memory is a severely limiting factor).

Disadvantages
1. Errors in recall (amount, frequency, and items used in preparation) may occur.
2. A 24-hour recall gives a poor idea of general diet and is specific only for that day.
3. Tendency to underestimate foods eaten on the part of the patient.
4. Method is time consuming and requires certain skills on the part of the practitioner.

Method 4: Usual Recalls

This method utilizes the patient's memory of all foods and beverages consumed during a usual period of consumption. Again, methods of preparation and additives that are used also are recalled. Open-ended questions still should be asked by the practioner, while intake again can be recorded on a blank piece of paper.

Advantages
1. Gives usual intake for a long period.
2. Inexpensive.
3. Suitable for use with illiterate patients as well as the aged (except when memory is a severely limiting factor.)

Disadvantages
1. Tends to be time consuming for the practitioner.
2. Errors in recall (amount, frequency, and items used in preparation) may occur.

Method 4a: Burke Method, Overall Pattern

24-Hour Recall

Advantages
1. Less time is needed by the clinician in questioning the patient.

Disadvantages
1. Small intakes usually are overreported by the patient while, at the same time, large intakes are underreported.
2. Frequent omissions of salad dressings, gravies, and all items used in food preparation can be expected.
3. Brief periods tend to offer poor estimate of patient's habitual intake.

Usual Frequency

Advantages
1. Probing is possible, which yields higher frequencies and more accurate information.

Disadvantages
1. Inaccurate recall may lead to inaccurate recording.

Method 4b: Burke Method, Food Preferences

Advantages
1. Can determine which foods patient consumes frequently.

Disadvantages
1. Frequent omissions can be expected.

Method 4c: Burke Method, 3-Day Record

Advantages
1. Gives more complete picture of what the patient ate.

Disadvantages
1. Resistance of subject to recording and remembering 3 days of food intake.

Method 5: Food Frequency Schedules or Questionnaires

This method allows the practitioner to obtain information on how many times per day, week, or month the patient eats specific foods or food groups. It originally was developed to allow a quick evaluation of menus and diet plans, and it can be used to help correlate other data that have been gathered to more accurately portray a patient's true eating pattern. Questions can be directed in particular areas that the clinician suspects may be deficient or excessive, or they may be more general.

Advantages	*Disadvantages*
1. The clinician can concentrate on items of interest.	1. Patients may have difficulty in estimating how often they ate a particular food.
2. Usual frequency can then be deduced.	2. Children and the aged often are not able to estimate intake accurately.
3. Compared with 7-day records, this correlates highly.	
4. Allows clinician to rapidly gather and analyze information.	

Method 5a: Computer Analysis

This method usually uses food frequency schedules (see Method 4) for evaluation.

Advantages	*Disadvantages*
1. Easy for the patient to read computer printout and does not take much time on the part of the practitioner.	1. No validity/reliability studies have been done to show the efficacy of this method.

Additional Questions

Along with the detailed analysis of the patient's dietary intake, the clinician should seek answers to the following questions:

Does the patient live alone and prepare his or her own meals?
How often does the patient shop for groceries?
What type of cooking facilities are available to the patient?
Is there frequent use of fad diets or monotonous diets?
Has the patient ever been placed on dietary restrictions?
Is there excess craving for:
    Sweets—candy, cake, ice cream
    Bread and butter
    Salt
    Coffee
    Fried food
    Alcohol
    "Junk food"
What foods are eaten every day?
What foods make the patient feel:
    Better
    Worse
What is the patient's favorite food?
Does the patient feel better after not eating at all?
Is there any reason to anticipate that the patient will be unable to eat for 10 days or longer?
Does the patient have an excessive appetite that is the result of:
    Nibbling all day long
    The inability to stop eating once he or she has started

Does the patient have poor appetite due to:
   Ill-fitting dentures
   Ageusia—lack or impaired sense of taste
   Loss of appetite
   Dysgeusia—impaired sense of taste
   Anosmia—lack of sense of smell
   Anorexia nervosa
   Chewing or swallowing problems
   Cultural or religious limitations
   Inability to eat more than one time per day
   Maintenance in intravenous fluids for more than 10 days
   Antibiotics or poor fluid intake
   Prolonged use of intravenous fluids
   Any adverse food and drug reactions
Does the patient drink milk or eat products that are made with milk? How much and how often?
Does the patient eat vegetables or fruit, or consume juices made from them? How much and how often?
Does the patient eat poultry, fish, eggs, or meat? How much and how often?
Does the patient cook with butter, margerine, salt, spices, oils, gravies, sugar, syrup, or other additives?

Interpretation of Data

Regardless of the method ultimately selected for obtaining a patient's dietary intake, the clinician must be prepared to evaluate the resultant information for nutritional sufficiency. Several methods are available for this evaluation, each offering distinct advantages and disadvantages.

Nutrient content, for example, can be evaluated by means of food composition tables or food groups. The former method is accurate but time consuming. The latter does not determine whether the patient's food intake is deficient in a particular nutrient, but it does provide a guideline to the general nutrient adequacy of the overall diet; it also may serve as a means of patient education for those who consume fewer servings in a particular food group than what is recommended. Both can be used in conjunction with recommended dietary allowances (RDAs).

In general, the major nutrients can be placed into a few distinct consumption classifications. The intake of vitamins A and C and folic acid, for instance, is considered to be the most variable in today's typical diet. These nutrients are not widely present in foods except for specific fruits and vegetables, so their ingestion is influenced most by conscious food choices and the seasons in which these foods are most available.

Riboflavin, calcium, and vitamin D, on the other hand, are dependent on the intake of milk and milk products, whereas thiamine, niacin, protein, phosphorous, calories, iron, and vitamins E, B_6, and B_{12} are more widely available and thus more easily ingested. Certain deficiencies in these nutrients are readily apparent from physical signs (see Fig. 2.3), whereas others must be uncovered through careful interpretation of dietary intake data.

Comparison of Dietary Interpretation Methods

Food Group Method

The quickest and most basic way to evaluate dietary intake is through a determination of the number of servings from each of the four basic food groups that the patient has consumed in a particular time period. This information then

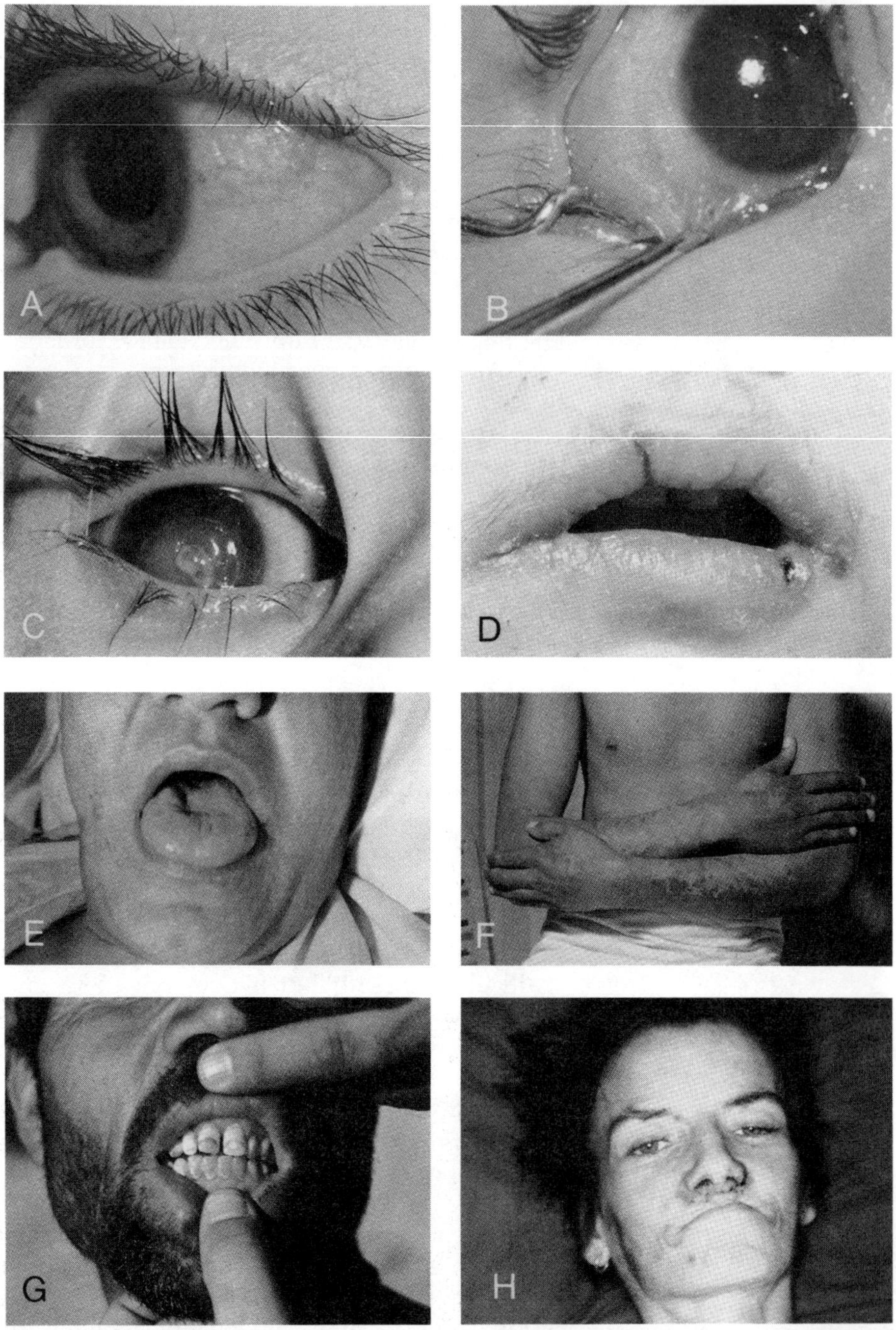

Figure 2.3. Deficiencies lead to physical signs. *A,* Bitot's spot in temporal interpalpebral fissure from a vitamin A deficiency. *B,* conjunctival and corneal xerosis from a vitamin A deficiency. *C,* keratomalacia from a vitamin A deficiency. *D,* cheilosis and angular stomatitis from a riboflavin deficiency. *E,* magenta tongue from a riboflavin deficiency. *F,* symmetrical dermatitis of pellagra from a niacin deficiency. *G,* early stage of fluorosis, with brown mottling most marked on central upper incisors. *H,* typical dermatosis stemming from patient's alcoholic cirrhosis signifies zinc deficiency. (From Shils ME, Young VR, eds. Modern nutrition in health and disease. 7th ed. Philadelphia: Lea & Febiger, 1988.)

is compared with the number of suggested servings from each of the various groups, and deficiencies are recorded. Shortcomings in nutrients like vitamins A and C, protein, calcium, riboflavin, and iron may be uncovered through this method, although the consumption of unusual foods may make this process more complex and somewhat unreliable.

Food Composition Tables

The patient's dietary intake can be assessed more accurately by calculating the amount of specific nutrients in each food or beverage that is consumed. This can be done by hand or with the aid of a computer (see Overview Of Computer Analysis below). Nutrient values for various foods and beverages can be obtained through a variety of sources, such as the United States Department of Agriculture, nutrition labels, and information from the appropriate manufacturers. Once the nutritional composition of each individual dietary item has been recorded, the practitioner then can determine the nutrient composition of the overall diet.

Recommended Dietary Allowances

Once nutritional composition is determined, it can be compared with the standard for evaluation of dietary intake: the recommended dietary allowance, or RDA. The practitioner must remember, however, that RDAs are set to include all members of a given population who might need increased amounts of a particular vitamin or mineral. RDAs, in addition, are not meant to be applied to individuals who are sick. These limitations, then, must be considered when RDAs are used to evaluate any specific patient's diet.

Overview of Computer Analysis

Clinicians always have used a variety of tools to help them analyze and evaluate the health of their patients. The advent of the microcomputer in recent years, however, has added a new and exciting dimension to this process. No longer are tedious manual systems necessary for complicated calculations or for various communication tasks. And, partly because of its often complex nature, nutritional assessment is one area that has benefited greatly by the widespread entry of computers into the health care arena.

With a computer, for example, the practitioner can store nutrient data on a file and then use it to quickly and accurately calculate the food intake of any patient. Methods for determining an individual's nutritional needs also can be stored, along with updated and relevant information about drugs, laboratory values, and anthropometric data; then, this information easily can be checked by the computer against a specific patient's nutrient profile. In addition, the computer can print out significant information on an individual for the practioner to provide to the patient for various educational purposes.

A vast array of software and hardware systems for computerized dietary evaluation are available today. Variables between them include the actual foods and nutrients stored in their files, the source of information they employ, the regularity and ease with which they can be updated, and the specific information that they eventually generate for the clinician's use. A careful examination of the practitioner's ultimate requirements, as well as the systems that are available, is necessary to ensure that an appropriate computerized dietary analysis system is obtained.

Computer System Selection

The process of selecting a microcomputer for dietary analysis is made easier when the specific tasks that will be expected of it are outlined in advance. What will it be used for? Who will use it? And how much training will these potential users require? Once this information is in hand, it can be compared with the specifications of systems currently on the market.

In order to do this properly, it is important to first identify the available systems and then define their strengths and limitations. What type of data base do they utilize? Are these data bases current and complete? How often will they be updated? What does the system do with the information it is given? How is it operated? Do manuals and instructions match the computer-literacy level of the intended users?

Information on available dietary computer systems can be obtained from a variety of sources. Details on finding them are provided in Chapter 7.

Because published tests on the validity of various data bases are rare, the evaluation of this critical characteristic usually involves a subjective appraisal on the part of the practitioner. The data's source and the reliability of the manufacturer are the most common measures utilized for this. The former is easiest for a clinician to determine, but the latter may have more bearing on the computer's ultimate effectiveness and ease of use. Determine whether the documentation and training that accompany the computer are adequate for those who will use it, for example; then examine the credentials of its developer to ascertain what—if any—nutritional training and background in designing a nutrient evaluation system may exist.

The examination of data base contents is another matter and one that is much easier to perform objectively. The completeness of a data base is measured by the number and types of foods it contains; the currency of it refers to how often it is updated. The size of these files can range from 50 to 15,000 foods and dietary components, and some researchers have determined that a data base should contain at least 3,000 in order to be considered valid. (The larger ones—which generally cost more to obtain and to maintain—may provide information on mixed dishes, brand name items, and fast foods; smaller data bases often focus on a specific type of food or select nutrients.)

In order to assess the data bases offered by various systems manufacturers, clinicians must first identify the nutrients that are used most often in their practice. An ability to change these data bases according to the practitioner's own needs—as well as evolving values in the profession—also is critical.

Finally, the operation and output of all available systems must be evaluated. Hardware requirements and their cost should be measured. (In some cases it may prove more efficient and effective to simply contract with a dietary analysis service, if one is offered nearby.) In addition, it is necessary to determine whether the systems offer a paper printout of the information they compile if the clinician intends to provide patients with evaluations and educational materials for further study.

Conclusion

Pencil and paper or a calculator can be used to help the clinician evaluate the dietary intake of a patient, but—just as it has in other fields—a computer will make the process more efficient and effective. Computers can store large amounts of up-to-date information, modify and analyze it, and then present it in a form that can be utilized easily by both the practitioner and the patient. Many professionals, once they have used a computer, find them to be invaluable. And they wonder how their work ever was accomplished before they installed one.

There is no perfect system yet offered for dietary evaluation, but there is a growing number that can be used to assist the health care professional in the complex process of nutrient analysis. The selection of a microcomputer and software for this purpose may be initially complex and time consuming, but it will most likely reap big rewards once a decision is made and the equipment is put into use.

Suggested Readings

Adelman MO, Dwyer JT. Computerized dietary analysis systems: a comparative view. Contin Educ 1883;83:421–428.

Anonymous. Experimental Nutrition: Validity of 24-hour dietary recalls. Nutr Rev 1976;34(10):310–311.

Beaton GH, Milner J. Sources of variance in 24-hour dietary recall data: implications for nutrition study design. Am J Clin Nutr 1979;32:2546–2559.

Cheraskin E. Psychodietetics. New York: Stein and Day, 1974.

Davidson SS, Passmore R, Brock JF, et al. Human nutrition and dietetics. New York: Churchill Livingstone, 1979.

el Lozy M. Programmable calculators in the field assessment of nutritional status. Am J Clin Nutr 1978;31:1718–1719.

Frank GC, Pelican S. Guidelines for selecting a dietary analysis system. Perspect Prac 1986;86:72–75.

Garn SM, Larkin FA. The problem with one-day dietary intakes. Ecol Food Nutr 1976;5:245.

Hodges RE. Nutrition in medical practice. Philadelphia: WB Saunders, 1980.

Hunt FI, Luke LS. Nutrient estimates from computerized questionnaires vs. 24-hour recall interviews. J Am Diet Assoc 1979;74:656–659.

Krause MV, Mahan LK. Food, nutrition, and diet therapy: a textbook of nutritional care. 7th ed. Philadelphia: WB Saunders, 1984.

Latanick MR, Gallagher-Allred CR. Appraisal of nutritional status. Columbus, Ohio: Department of Family Medicine, The Ohio State University, 1980.

Madden JP. Validity of the 24-hour recall. J Am Diet Assoc 1976;68:143.

Mo A, Peckos PS. Computers in a dietary study. J Am Diet Assoc 1971;59:111–115.

Roberge AG, Sevigny J. Dietary intake data: usefullness and limitations. Prog Food Nutr Sci 1984;8:27–42.

Seltzer MH, Bastidas J. Instant nutritional assessment. Parent Ent Nutr 1979;3(3):157–159.

Shapiro LR. Streamlining and implementing nutritional assessment: the dietary approach. J Am Diet Assoc 1979;75(3):230–237.

Shils ME, Young VR, eds. Modern nutrition in health and disease. 7th ed. Philadelphia: Lea & Febiger, 1988.

Todd KS, Hudes M, Calloway, DH. Food intake measurement: problems and approaches. Am J Clin Nutr 1983;37:139–146.

3

Anthropometric and Body Composition Assessments

There are a number of body measurements that are sensitive to dietary intake and thus can be used to help evaluate the nutritional status of the patient. These measurements are divided into two basic categories: anthropometric assessment and body composition assessment. Various techniques are available to the practitioner who wishes to undertake these processes, and the more prominent among them are discussed fully in this chapter.

Of the two complementary assessment systems, anthropometric measurements are the most easily utilized. In order to ensure that thorough testing and accurate evaluation will be accomplished through them, it is necessary to obtain data on the following: height, weight, body frame, triceps and/or subscapular skinfold, arm circumference, arm muscle circumference, and arm muscle area. Tests to obtain this data can be performed quickly, and necessary equipment is both available and inexpensive.

In turn, these measurements can be used to evaluate:

1. The amount of body fat;
2. The amount of muscle mass;
3. The degree of protein-calorie malnutrition;
4. The degree of obesity;
5. The changes in nutritional status that may occur over a period of time, or because of special circumstances (e.g., hospitalization);
6. The continuing health status of the patient.

Undertaking this measurement process will add only a small amount of time to any comprehensive nutritional evaluation. And, from this initial examination on, these measurements also can be used to track the patient's continuing progress. A flexible steel or nonstretch fiberglass tape and skinfold calipers are used for the physical examinations; various tables and charts are then consulted for the appropriate correlations.

Although standard height/weight tables used in conjunction with anthropometric measurements will present the clinician with critical insight into a patient's overall condition, it is important to remember that they usually are based on wide-ranging averages for the population at-large. The precise evaluation of an individual's actual body composition, on the other hand, will give the practitioner more exact information on that patient's major structural components (i.e., muscles, bones, and fat).

A body composition analysis, therefore, offers an explicit look at the relative quality of a specific patient's body weight. This leads to additional insight into the patient's total nutritional status and can be accomplished by several methods. Three of them—underwater weighing, neutron activation, and bioelectric impedance—are discussed extensively in the following pages.

In all, the two assessment procedures go hand in hand during any complete evaluation of a patient's nutritional status. The information they reveal jointly and alone, in conjunction with other clinical evaluations and case histories, will help the practitioner to accurately pinpoint specific dietary deficiencies and excesses. Eventually, this data will help the clinician determine a correct therapeutic course of action.

Height and Weight

Accurate measurement of body weight and height can be accomplished quite easily, and they will prove to be of tremendous use in the assessment of nutritional status. Because verbally expressed reports on height and weight by patients themselves tend to be inaccurate, however, the practitioner should perform these measurements individually for each patient. And since these are among the most critical measurements that the clinician will make during an assessment, they must be performed consistently.

Adult height should be measured against a flat surface while the patient— barefoot or wearing socks—stands erect with feet together and head level; length then should be recorded to the nearest quarter-inch. Children under 3 years should be measured for crown-heel length while in the recumbent position. To accomplish this most accurately, it is necessary to lay the child on a ruled board that has an attached piece of wood on one end and a movable piece at the other. Make sure the child is stretched out with the top of the head against the stationary end and the feet flat against the movable end. Length, as noted from the board, then should be plotted on a growth chart.

For weight, the practitioner should use reliable lever-balance or beam balance scales that have been periodically calibrated for accuracy. The patient should wear light clothing and no shoes, and subsequent measurements always should be taken at the same time of day. Adult weight should be recorded to the nearest half-pound, and infants should be recorded at the nearest quarter-pound. For adults, regular weight measurements are particularly critical if chronic illness is present; for children, they can offer an early indication of growth problems and nutritional deficiencies.

The patient's weight then should be evaluated in relation to his or her height by use of various norms. Children are assessed by comparing their height and weight with the total population at similar ages, which is a measurement usually expressed in percentiles. Straight height-weight tables often are used for adults, but there are various limitations inherent in this method. Much more relevant information can be obtained by utilizing a chart showing desirable weights according to height and body frame (see Table 3.1). Then, the resultant data can be used more effectively after other anthropometric measurements are conducted.

Determination of Wrist Circumference

The measurement of wrist circumference is used to determine the body frame size of the patient. Once this information is gathered, the practitioner can more accurately evaluate the patient's weight in relation to height.

Table 3.1
Ideal Height/Weight Tables[a]
This updated data is for patients aged 25 to 59; it assumes male patients are wearing 5 pounds of indoor clothing, female patients are wearing 3 pounds, and both are wearing 1-inch heels. (From the Metropolitan Life Insurance Company, 1983.)

Height	Men			Women		
	Small Frame	Medium Frame	Large Frame	Small Frame	Medium Frame	Large Frame
4 ft 10 in	—	—	—	102–111	109–121	118–131
4 ft 11 in	—	—	—	103–113	111–123	120 134
5 ft	—	—	—	104–115	113–126	122–137
5 ft 1 in	—	—	—	106–118	115–129	125–140
5 ft 2 in	128–134	131–141	138–150	108–121	118–132	128–143
5 ft 3 in	130–136	133–143	140–153	111–124	121–135	131–147
5 ft 4 in	132–138	135–145	142–156	114–127	124–138	134–151
5 ft 5 in	134–140	137–148	144–160	117–130	127–141	137–155
5 ft 6 in	136–142	139–151	146–164	120–133	130–144	140–159
5 ft 7 in	138–145	142–154	149–168	123–136	133–147	143–163
5 ft 8 in	140–148	145–157	152–172	126–139	136–150	146–167
5 ft 9 in	142–151	148–160	155–176	129–142	139–153	149–170
5 ft 10 in	144–154	151–163	158–180	132–145	142–156	152–173
5 ft 11 in	148–157	154–166	161–184	135–148	145–159	155–176
6 ft	149–160	157–170	164–188	138–151	148–162	158–179
6 ft 1 in	152–164	160–174	168–192	—	—	—
6 ft 2 in	155–168	164–178	172–197	—	—	—
6 ft 3 in	158–172	167–182	176–202	—	—	—
6 ft 4 in	162–176	171–187	181–207	—	—	—

[a]Ages 25 through 59, for 5 lb of indoor clothing for men and 3 lb of indoor clothing for women, and 1-in heels for both. Data from The Metropolitan Life Insurance Company, 1983.

Method of Measuring Wrist Circumference

1. A linear tape should be placed around the smallest part of the wrist distal to the styloid processes of the radius and ulna (see Fig. 3.1).
2. After this is completed, the clinician can use the resultant data to determine the body frame size (see Table 3.2).
3. When this information is gathered, the practitioner can refer back to Table 3.1 for the patient's ideal body weight.
4. To then obtain data on the percentage of ideal body weight, the clinician can use the following formula:

$$\frac{\text{current weight}}{\text{ideal weight}} \times 100$$

For example, a woman 5'5" with a small frame weighing 132 pounds is found to be 10% overweight using the following formula:

$$\frac{132}{120} \times 100 = \frac{1320}{120} = 110\%$$

or 10% over the ideal weight.

Body Mass Index

The practitioner may find the Body Mass Index (or BMI) to be another useful measurement in the overall clinical assessment of a patient's nutritional status. The BMI does not measure a patient's fat compartment directly, but it does correlate weight and height in order to estimate overall fat stores.

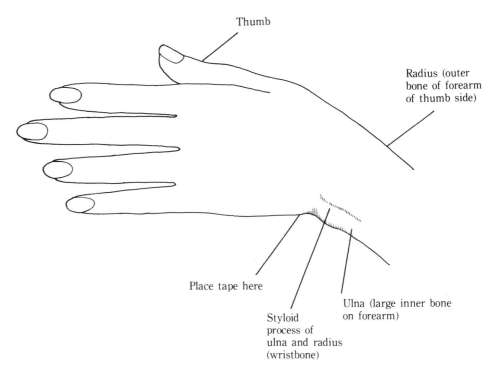

Figure 3.1. Measuring wrist circumference. The patient's wrist circumference should be measured using linear tape placed around the smallest part of the wrist distal to the styloid processes of the radius and ulna.

BMI is body weight divided by a power of height. The assessment formula is as follows:

$$BMI = weight(kg)/height(m)^2 \times 100$$

It is suggested that BMI for normal men and women should be in the range of 19 to 27. For infants and children, average BMI values change with age; they begin at 13 at birth, reach a peak of 18 at about 1 year, and a nadir of 15 at about 6 years.

The practitioner should remember that the BMI may be affected by hydration status, and it may classify some very muscular individuals as obese when in reality they are not. These problems are minor, though, and the BMI can prove especially useful when it is considered in conjunction with skinfold measurements in order to estimate total body fat. Alone, it may help the clinician estimate the patient's fat compartment if skinfold measurements cannot be made for any reason; it must be noted, however, that the BMI by itself will not provide a completely accurate evaluation of body composition.

Measurement of Triceps Skinfold

Triceps skinfold measurement is a practical, inexpensive, and objective way to assist the clinician in a total assessment of the patient's nutritional status. In order to measure the triceps skinfold, an instrument called a caliper must be used (see Fig. 3.2).

The triceps skinfold is a way to measure the thickness of the subcutaneous fat ring. Because a thin ring on a muscular arm may contain as much fat as a thicker ring around a small muscle, the triceps skinfold measrement cannot be used as the sole tool for evaluating the body's fat reserves. Nonetheless, the clinician

Table 3.2
Body Frame Type
To determine frame type, the clinician should use height without shoes and inches for wrist size. The wrist is measured distal to styloid process of radius and ulna at smallest circumference. (Reproduced with permission from Peter G. Lidner, M.D., 1973.)

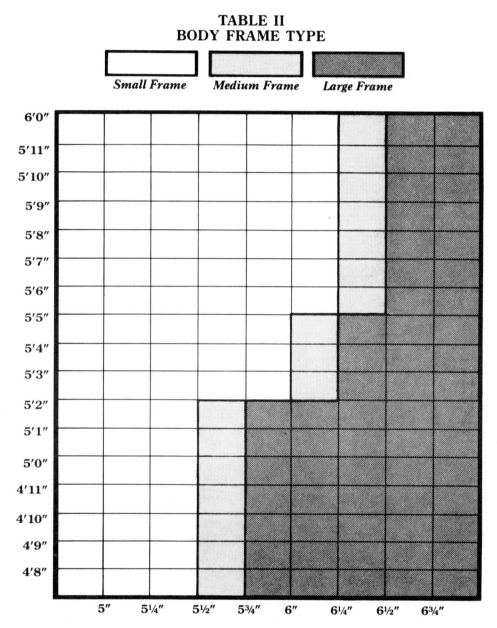

TABLE II
BODY FRAME TYPE

Small Frame   Medium Frame   Large Frame

certainly can use it as one tool to evaluate body fat and calorie stores. And triceps skinfold measurement often will correlate with other measurements of body fat.

Skinfold thickness can be measured at several sites, but the measurement usually is taken over the triceps muscle because the most complete standards and the best assessment methods have been developed for this site. (Gross obesity, however, will increase measurement error.) The amount of body fat then can be evaluated against population standards that are age and sex appropriate (see Table 3.3) to determine the degree of either obesity or protein-calorie malnutrition.

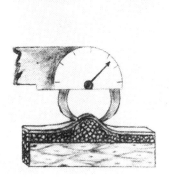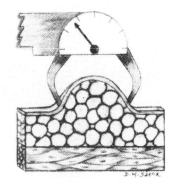

Figure 3.2. Skinfold calipers. Thickness of the patient's subcutaneous fat tissue should be measured by means of skinfold calipers; *left*, calipers respond to appropriate weight; *right*, measurement of an obese individual. (From Krause MV, Mahan LK. Food, nutrition and diet therapy: a textbook of nutritional care. 7th ed. Philadelphia: WB Saunders, 1984.)

Method Of Measurement

Triceps skinfold should be measured on the right arm, unless arm edema or paralysis is present. If possible, the patient should be standing erect with arm and shoulder bare; otherwise, the patient should be sitting erect. The arm should be held vertically, and not be resting on any surface.

Because fat thickness at the triceps muscle will not be uniform, the measurement always should be taken at a specific point. Ideally, this will be the midpoint of the arm—between the acromion and olecranon process, on the posterior side—which first must be determined and marked. This can be accomplished by using a flexible metric tape to measure the upper arm between the aforementioned reference points.

After the measuring point is marked, the practitioner should fully separate the thumb and index finger of his or her left hand, grasp a full skinfold (at least two thicknesses), and then raise that fold far enough to allow the muscle to fall back to the bone. The remaining skinfold and subcutaneous fat is held lightly, calipers are placed on the fold at a point 1 cm below the clinician's fingers (see Fig. 3.3), and a reading is taken to the nearest half-millimeter. The skinfold then is released. Accurate assessments are best obtained by measuring the skinfold three times—completely releasing the caliper and grasp each time—and computing an average.

It may, however, be more desirable to measure skinfold below the scapula (subscapular). This measurement can be performed in much the same manner as that described for the triceps skinfold (see Fig. 3.4).

Comparison Of Calipers

A caliper suitable for measuring skinfold thickness will offer a standard contact surface, or "pinch area," of between 20 and 40 mm; it also will exert a constant pressure at all jaw separation points. Several brands of calipers are available for measuring the patient's skinfold. A comparison of two follows:

Type of Calipers	Advantages	Disadvantages
Lange	1. Accurate. 2. Can be used with obese patients.	1. More expensive. 2. Relatively bulky for field work.

Table 3.3
Right Arm Skinfold Averages
This chart shows the average right arm skinfold and selected percentiles for adults by age and sex, 1960–62. (From Stout HW, Duncan A. Skinfolds, body girths, biacromial diameter, and selected anthropometric indices of adults: United States 1960–1962. Vital and Health Statistics Series 11, National Health Survey No. 35. Washington, DC: United States Department of Health, Education and Welfare, Public Health Service, 1970.)

Sex, Average and Percentile	18–79 Years	18–24 Years	25–34 Years	35–44 Years	45–54 Years	55–64 Years	65–74 Years	Total 75–79 Years
MEN				Measurement in Centimeters[b]				
Average right arm skinfold	1.3	1.1	1.4	1.4	1.3	1.2	1.2	1.1
Percentile[a]								
99	4.1	3.7	4.5	4.0	3.8	3.3	3.2	3.0
95	2.8	2.6	3.3	2.9	2.8	2.4	2.7	2.0
90	2.3	2.4	2.6	2.4	2.2	2.0	2.2	1.7
80	1.8	1.7	2.0	1.9	1.8	1.6	1.7	1.5
70	1.5	1.3	1.6	1.6	1.5	1.4	1.4	1.3
60	1.3	1.1	1.4	1.4	1.3	1.3	1.3	1.1
50	1.1	0.9	1.2	1.2	1.1	1.2	1.1	1.0
40	1.0	0.8	1.0	1.1	1.0	1.0	1.0	0.9
30	0.8	0.7	0.8	1.0	0.9	0.9	0.8	0.8
20	0.7	0.6	0.7	0.8	0.7	0.8	0.7	0.7
10	0.6	0.5	0.5	0.6	0.6	0.6	0.6	0.6
5	0.5	0.5	0.5	0.5	0.5	0.5	0.5	0.5
1	0.4	0.4	0.4	0.4	0.4	0.4	0.4	0.4
WOMEN								
Average right arm skinfold	2.2	1.8	2.1	2.3	2.4	2.5	2.4	2.0
Percentile[a]								
99	4.6	4.3	4.7	4.6	4.8	4.7	4.7	3.9
95	3.8	3.2	3.7	3.9	4.0	4.0	3.6	3.3
90	3.4	2.8	3.2	3.5	3.6	3.7	3.4	3.1
80	3.0	2.4	2.8	3.0	3.2	3.2	3.0	2.7
70	2.6	2.1	2.4	2.7	2.8	2.9	2.7	2.5
60	2.4	2.0	2.2	2.5	2.6	2.7	2.5	2.3
50	2.2	1.7	2.0	2.3	2.4	2.5	2.4	2.2
40	2.0	1.6	1.9	2.1	2.2	2.3	2.2	2.0
30	1.8	1.5	1.7	1.8	2.0	2.1	2.0	1.7
20	1.6	1.3	1.5	1.6	1.8	1.9	1.7	1.4
10	1.3	1.1	1.2	1.4	1.5	1.6	1.5	1.0
5	1.1	0.9	1.0	1.2	1.2	1.4	1.2	0.7
1	0.8	0.6	0.7	1.0	0.8	1.0	0.8	0.3

[a]Measurement below which the indicated percentage of persons in the given age group falls.
[b]To convert to millimeters multiply values by 10.

McGaw	1. Lightweight. 2. Less expensive.	1. Maximal scale is 40 mm. 2. Usefulness is limited for obese patients.

Other measurement tools include the Harpenden calipers and the US AMRNL calipers.

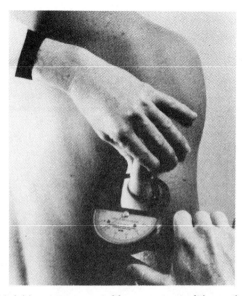

Figure 3.3. Triceps skinfold measurement. Measurement of the patient's triceps skinfold is made at a point over the triceps muscle, midway between the acromion process and olecranon process. (From Krause MV, Mahan LK. Food, nutrition and diet therapy: a textbook of nutritional care. 7th ed. Philadelphia: W.B. Saunders, 1984.)

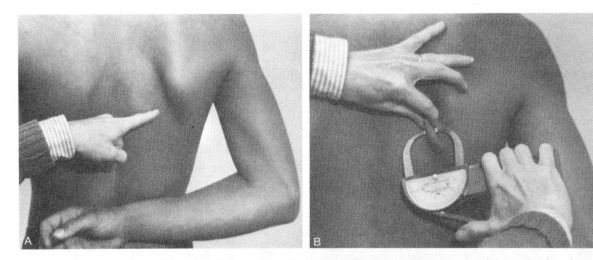

Figure 3.4. Subscapular skinfold measurement. Measurement of the patient's subscapular skinfold is made at the point shown in the photo at *left*, in the manner shown in the photo at *right*. (From Krause MV, Mahan LK. Food, nutrition and diet therapy: a textbook of nutritional care. 7th ed. Philadelphia: W.B. Saunders, 1984.)

Measurement of Arm Circumference

If more information is needed, additional anthropometric evaluations can be performed. Because poor muscle development and muscle wasting are features common to all forms of protein-calorie malnutrition—particularly in early childhood—a direct measurement of arm circumference and arm muscle mass can prove to be a useful and practical way to assess any deficiencies.

Method Of Measurement

As with the previous measurements, the patient's right arm should be used if possible (see Fig. 3.5). After the patient's forearm is bent across his or her stomach, the clinician should locate the midpoint between acromion process at

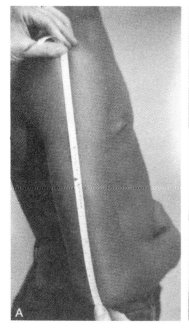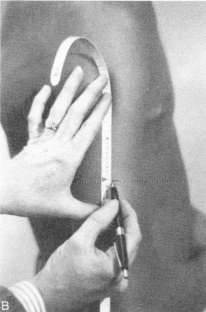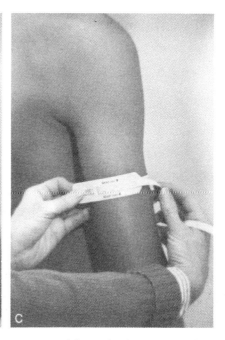

Figure 3.5. Arm circumference measurement. Measurement of the patient's arm circumference is made by first determining the midpoint between acromion process at shoulder and olecranon process at elbow as shown in photo at *left*; this is then marked as shown in *center* photo; measurements are taken in centimeters as shown in photo at *right*. (From Krause MV, Mahan LK. Food, nutrition and diet therapy: a textbook of nutritional care. 7th ed. Philadelphia: WB Saunders, 1984.)

shoulder and olecranon process at elbow. This should be marked, and a flexible steel or nonstretch fiberglass tape can be used for measurement while the patient's arm is hanging relaxed. The tape should be held firmly but gently so there is no compression of the soft tissue. Then, results can be compared with sex-specific norms (see Table 3.4).

Determination of Arm Muscle Circumference and Area

The measurement of the arm muscle circumference is considered a sensitive index in assessing the body's protein stores. In addition, the area of the cross-sectional arm muscle also can be estimated. Both measurements are particularly useful in determining protein-calorie malnutrition. The second measurement also is quite helpful in the assessment of children, as arm muscle area changes less frequently with age than does arm muscle circumference. However, the

Table 3.4
Arm Circumference.
This chart shows arm circumference for adult men and women. (Adapted from O'Brien and Shelton, 1941; Hertzberg R. 1963.)

Sex	Arm Circumference (cm)				
	Standard	90% Standard	80% Standard	70% Standard	60% Standard
Male	29.3	26.3	23.4	20.5	17.6
Female	28.5	25.7	22.8	20.0	17.1

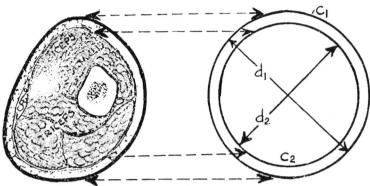

Figure 3.6. Determining upper arm measurments. The patient's upper arm area, upper arm muscle area, and upper arm fat area can be determined through use of upper arm circumference and triceps skinfold measurement as described in the text. (From Krause MV, Mahan LK. Food, nutrition and diet therapy: a textbook of nutritional care. 7th ed. Philadelphia: WB Saunders Company, 1984.)

clinician must take into account that arm muscle measurement only can be estimated because the thickness of the humerus is not taken into account and upper arms are not perfectly round as the formula presumes. In addition, the fat compressibility varies, with greater compressibility occurring in females and the obese than in males and the nonobese.

The clinician can determine both arm muscle circumference and arm muscle area from the measurements of arm circumference and triceps fatfold. This can be done through the use of nomograms as developed by Gurney or through the use of mathematical formulas.

Calculation by Mathematical Formula

Measurement of upper arm circumference and triceps skinfold in millimeters first must be obtained in order to calculate arm muscle and fat area by formula (see Fig. 3.6). These measurements then can be used to estimate upper arm area, upper arm muscle area, and upper arm fat area by use of the following:

C1 = upper arm circumference
T = triceps skinfold
A = upper arm area
M = upper arm muscle area
F = upper arm fat area
π = 3.14

$$A\ (mm^2) = \frac{\pi}{4} \times d1^2 \text{ where } d1 = \frac{C1}{\pi}$$
$$M\ (mm^2) = \frac{(C1 - \pi T)^2}{4\pi} = \frac{(C1 - \pi T)^2}{12.56}$$
$$F\ (mm^2) = A - M$$

In addition, standards for arm muscle circumference and arm muscle area can be compared with the results that have been obtained (see Tables 3.5 and 3.6).

Calculation Using Nomograms

Arm area and muscle area also can be determined through the use of nomograms. In order to do so, the practitioner should follow these steps:

1. Measure the patient's triceps fatfold in millimeters.
2. Measure the patient's midupper arm circumference in centimeters.

Table 3.5
Arm Muscle Circumference
This chart shows the standards for arm muscle circumference of males and females, by various age groups, in centimeters. The percentiles are derived from data obtained on all white subjects in the United States Ten-State Nutritional Survey of 1968–70. (Adapted from Frisancho A. Triceps skinfold and upper arm muscle size norms for assessment of nutritional status. Am J Clin Nutr 1974;27:1052.)

Age	Male					Female				
	5th	15th	50th	85th	95th	5th	15th	50th	85th	95th
0–5 mo.	8.1	9.6	10.6	12.5	13.3	8.6	9.2	10.4	11.5	12.6
6 17 mo.	10.0	10.8	12.3	13.7	14.6	9.7	10.2	11.7	12.8	13.5
1½–2½ yr.	11.1	11.7	12.7	13.8	14.6	10.5	11.2	12.5	14.0	14.6
2½–3½	11.4	12.1	13.2	14.5	15.2	10.8	11.6	12.8	13.8	14.3
3½–4½	11.8	12.4	13.5	15.1	15.7	11.4	12.0	13.2	14.6	15.2
4½–5½	12.1	13.0	14.1	15.6	16.6	11.9	12.4	13.8	15.1	16.0
5½–6½	12.7	13.4	14.6	15.9	16.7	12.1	12.9	14.0	15.5	16.5
6½–7½	13.0	13.7	15.1	16.4	17.3	12.3	13.2	14.6	16.2	17.5
7½–8½	13.8	14.4	15.8	17.4	18.5	12.9	13.8	15.1	16.8	18.6
8½–9½	13.8	14.3	16.1	18.2	20.0	13.6	14.3	15.7	17.6	19.3
9½–10½	14.2	15.2	16.8	18.6	20.2	13.9	14.7	16.3	18.2	19.6
10½–11½	15.0	15.8	17.4	19.4	21.1	14.0	15.2	17.1	19.5	20.9
11½–12½	15.3	16.3	18.1	20.7	22.1	15.0	16.1	17.9	20.0	21.2
12½–13½	15.9	16.9	19.5	22.4	24.2	15.5	16.5	18.5	20.6	22.5
13½–14½	16.7	18.2	21.1	23.4	26.5	16.6	17.5	19.3	22.1	23.4
14½–15½	17.3	18.5	22.0	25.2	27.1	16.3	17.3	19.5	22.0	23.2
15½–16½	18.6	20.5	22.9	26.0	28.1	17.1	17.8	20.0	22.7	26.0
16½–17½	20.6	21.7	24.5	27.1	29.0	17.1	17.7	19.6	22.3	24.1
17½–24½	21.7	23.2	25.8	28.6	30.5	17.0	18.3	20.5	22.9	25.3
24½–34½	22.0	24.1	27.0	29.5	31.5	17.7	28.9	21.3	24.5	27.2
34½–44½	22.2	23.9	27.0	30.0	31.8	18.0	19.2	21.6	25.0	27.9

3. Select the appropriate table (see Figs. 3.7 and 3.8), then use a ruler to connect the values measured in Steps 1 and 2 as represented on the outside two columns of the table that has been selected. Determine the arm muscle circumference and the arm muscle area by noting where the ruler crosses the center column.

4. If the values are either too low or too high, the nomogram cannot be used. In that case, arm muscle circumference must be calculated instead by use of the formula method.

Comparison of Anthropometric Assessment Methods

Method 1: Height-Weight Indices

Height and weight are measured:

Advantages
1. Easily performed by clinician in the office.
2. Weight changes can be monitored.

Disadvantages
1. Height and weight alone are quite inaccurate in measurement of protein-calorie malnutrition.
2. Somewhat more accurate is the weight to height squared index.

Table 3.6
Arm Muscle Area
  This chart shows the standards for arm muscle area of males and females, by various age groups, in square centimeters. The percentiles are derived from data obtained on all white subjects in the United States Ten-State Nutritional Survey of 1968–70. (Adapted from Frisancho A. Triceps skinfold and upper arm muscle size norms for assessment of nutritional status. Am J Clin Nutr 1974;27:1052.)

Age	Male					Female				
	5th	15th	50th	85th	95th	5th	15th	50th	85th	95th
0–5 mo.	52.2	70.3	89.2	124.4	141.4	59.1	67.0	86.6	105.8	127.2
6–17 mo.	79.1	92.8	120.1	150.0	169.0	75.6	82.1	108.4	130.4	146.0
1½–2½ yr.	97.8	108.2	128.4	152.5	168.6	88.5	99.1	124.1	155.1	169.3
2½–3½	102.7	116.3	138.4	167.0	184.2	92.8	106.8	129.8	151.6	162.8
3½–4½	110.6	122.4	145.1	180.5	197.3	104.0	114.3	139.0	169.3	182.8
4½–5½	117.1	134.2	157.9	193.0	219.3	111.9	122.7	151.6	182.5	204.5
5½–6½	127.5	143.5	170.0	201.9	222.0	116.3	133.3	156.3	190.2	217.4
6½–7½	134.2	148.5	181.5	215.2	238.6	121.3	138.4	170.0	209.6	243.3
7½–8½	150.6	164.7	198.7	239.8	272.9	132.2	151.3	181.8	223.9	275.8
8½–9½	152.2	163.7	207.4	264.5	318.8	147.3	162.5	195.5	247.7	197.8
9½–10½	160.8	183.2	223.9	275.3	323.9	152.8	172.7	211.5	263.7	306.6
10½–11½	180.1	198.7	240.6	300.0	354.4	155.1	184.2	233.5	301.8	348.6
11½–12½	187.4	212.6	260.3	340.1	390.2	178.1	205.2	255.8	318.3	358.2
12½–13½	201.2	227.3	301.3	399.8	466.1	190.5	217.8	271.1	338.2	401.4
13½–14½	223.1	264.5	354.4	435.8	560.1	218.6	243.0	295.2	388.3	435.8
14½–15½	237.5	272.9	386.7	506.0	582.6	212.6	238.7	303.1	383.8	427.9
15½–16½	274.1	333.1	418.4	536.3	626.6	231.6	251.0	319.8	409.6	538.6
16½–17½	337.3	374.3	477.1	582.6	671.3	231.6	250.2	305.8	396.8	461.2
17½–24½	374.8	427.3	531.5	652.9	741.1	228.9	267.9	334.1	416.4	508.9
24½–34½	383.7	463.4	580.2	691.2	791.8	248.6	285.6	360.6	277.2	588.9
34½–44½	393.8	456.3	582.0	718.3	804.1	256.6	292.6	372.4	499.1	619.5

Method 2: Triceps Skinfold

Body fat and calorie stores are measured:

Advantages	*Disadvantages*
1. Easily performed in the clinician's office. 2. Accurate in the measurement of body fat. 3. If average is under or over the standard, a diagnosis of either obesity or malnutrition can be made.	1. Sometimes may prove insufficient in and of itself.

Method 3: Arm Circumference

Protein and muscle mass are measured:

Advantages	*Disadvantages*
1. Easily performed by practitioner's assistant.	1. Only measures severe protein-calorie malnutrition. 2. Cannot be used to assess moderate changes in protein stores.

Method 4: Arm Muscle Circumference

Protein and muscle mass are measured:

Advantages
1. More accurate estimate can be made with this measurement in determining protein-calorie malnutrition.

Disadvantages
1. This measurement is only an estimate because the thickness of the humerus is not taken into account.
2. No patient's upper arm is perfectly round according to the formula.

Method 5: Arm Muscle Area

Protein and muscle mass are measured:

Advantages
1. More complete assessment of nutritional status.
2. A more sensitive index for measuring protein status in children.
3. Can be used to follow patient's progress to medical and nutritional therapies.

Disadvantages
1. This measurement is an estimate for the same reasons listed in Method 4.

Overview of Body Composition Assessment Methods

Research into various methods that could be used for the indirect determination of body composition have been conducted for nearly 50 years. Several of those that are available today permit the practitioner to accurately evaluate the patient's major structural components: muscle, bone, and fat. However, unlike anthropometic measurements—in which evalations are based on statistical averages—body composition analysis reveals the relative composition and quality of a specific patient's body weight. When they can be performed in conjunction with anthropometric measurements, therefore, the results will be much more revealing than those from anthropometric evaluations alone.

The three major structural components of the human body vary according to sex, however, and so it is still very important to compare a patient's body composition with the correct statistical model. The theoretical "Reference Man" and "Reference Woman" proposed by Dr. Albert Behnke (see Fig. 3.9) usually are used for this purpose. They are based on the average dimensions derived from measuring thousands of individuals in widespread studies and so are considered quite repesentative for these purposes.

Underwater Weighing

One of the most popular and precise techniques for measuring body composition is called underwater or hydrostatic weighing. Based on the Archimedean principles relating the weight of matter with the volume of water it displaces, this method involves weighing a patient first in the air and then while he or she

NOMOGRAM FOR DETERMINATION OF ARM MUSCLE CIRCUMFERENCE AND ARM MUSCLE AREA

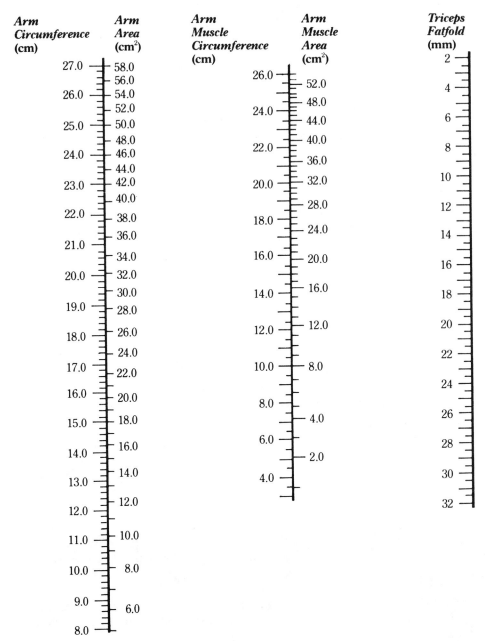

Figures 3.7 and 3.8. Nomogram for determination of arm muscle circumference and arm muscle area. To calculate muscle circumference and area, lay a ruler between the appropriate values for *arm circumference* and *triceps fatfold* on the outside columns and then read off the *muscle circumference* and *muscle area* from the middle line. (From Gurney J, Jelliffe D. Arm anthropometry in nutritional assessment: nomogram for rapid calculation of muscle circumference and cross-sectional muscle and fat areas. Am J Clin Nutr 1973;26:912.)

is submerged. The density of the body and the percentage of body fat can be calculated from a determination of these two variables.

Under this method, the patient is first weighed carefully on an accurate balance scale. When he or she is seated on a lightweight chair suspended from a scale, both patient and scale are submerged completely in water maintained at

TABLE VIII
NOMOGRAM FOR DETERMINATION OF ARM MUSCLE CIRCUMFERENCE AND ARM MUSCLE AREA.

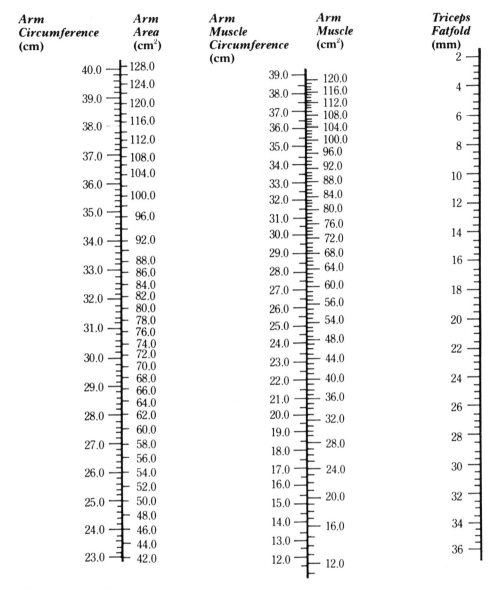

Figures 3.7 and 3.8 continued.

approximately 95°F. (Water temperature is recorded in order to correct for the density at the weighing temperature.) The patient forcibly exhales as his or her head is lowered beneath the surface of the water, and then the breath is held for 5 to 10 seconds while weight is recorded. This is repeated a dozen times, with the last two or three averaged in order to obtain a proper reading.

The following can be determined from these measurements:

1. Body volume = the difference between body weight in air and in water when any necessary correction for water temperature is applied.

2. $$\text{Density} = \frac{\text{Mass}}{\text{Volume}}$$

3. $$\text{Percentage of body fat} = \frac{495}{\text{Density}} - 450$$

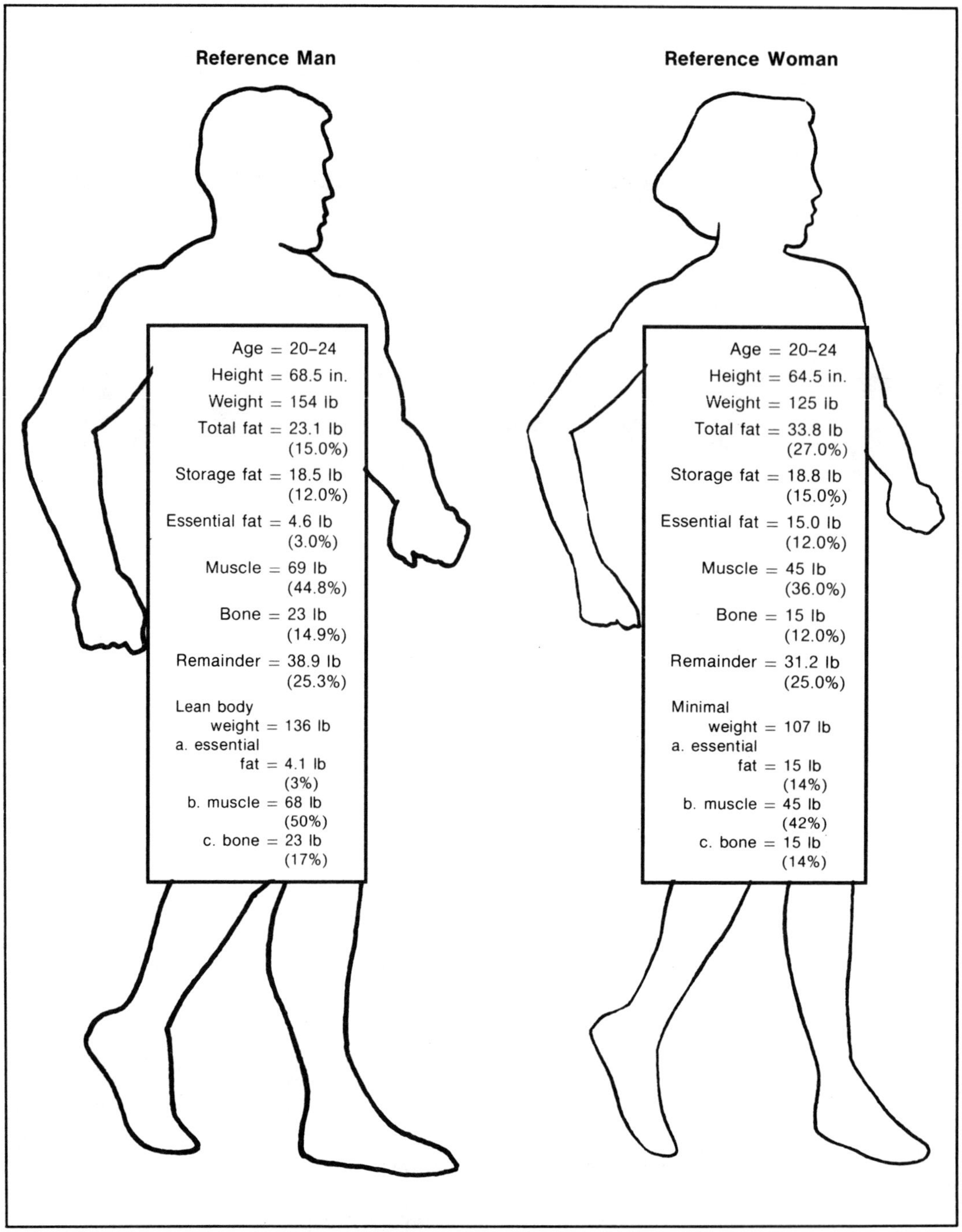

Figure 3.9. Reference man and woman. Theoretical models for a reference man and woman were originally developed by Behnke. (From McArdle WD, Katch FI, Katch VL. Exercise physiology: energy, nutrition, and human performance. 2nd ed. Philadelphia: Lea & Febiger, 1986.)

4. Fat weight = (Percentage of fat/100) × body weight
5. Lean body weight = body weight − fat weight

Neutron Activation

Total body neutron activation analysis provides the clinician with a way to measure even more elements in the patient's body that help to comprise nutritional status. These include calcium, sodium, chloride, phosphorous, and nitrogen. Sys-

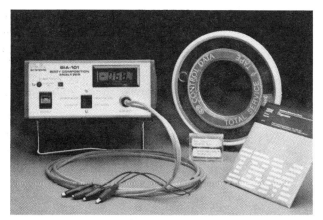

Figure 3.10. Computerized body composition. The RJL Systems BIA-101 can measure total body water, lean body mass, and total body fat with reproducible results. (From RJL Systems.)

tems created for in vivo neutron activation studies will deliver a beam of fast neutrons to the patient's body; they are captured by these target elements and the data obtained by recording the resultant radiation enables identification and determination of activity levels by means of a standard gamma spectrographic analysis.

Total body calcium and total body nitrogen are two of the more useful measurements obtained through the use of this method. The former allows the practitioner to estimate bone mineral mass, and the latter permits estimation of muscle and nonmuscle mass; together with body mass, these can be used to calculate body fat.

Bioelectric Impedance

Bioelectric impedance analysis (or BIA) is a method for estimating the percentage of body fat by using an instrument that introduces a tiny electrical current into the patient's body and then reads the resistance to that current. Portable BIA units can combine an impedance analyzer with either a briefcase-sized computer of its own or an IBM-compatible computer disk, both of which are programmed with equations for specific populations (see Fig. 3.10).

Under this method, electrocardiogram electrodes are attached to the patient's wrist and ankle. Lean tissue contains most of the water and electrolytes in the body, so the less electrical resistance that is measured the more lean tissue is present. A full "Body Composition Profile" then can be generated from the data that is derived, as well as exercise recommendations (see Fig. 3.11). However, it must be remembered that a variety of factors—including use of diuretics, alcohol consumption, the presence of edema, ascites, heart failure, and exercise with sweating or dehydration—can affect the resistance measured by certain systems and render their analysis inaccurate.

Comparison of Body Composition Assessment Methods

Method 1: Underwater Weighing

Body density and body fat percentage are measured:

Advantages	*Disadvantages*
1. Proven to be a valid method for determining body fat content.	1. Available only in specialized settings.

```
               BODY  COMPOSITION  PROFILE
##############################################################
                  My  Company  Name
##############################################################
                                              August 25, 1988
                                                      6:15 am

                  James  Michaels
                 Patient ID No. ABC-007

Sex : male                       Age : 28
Height :  70.0 in                Weight : 190.0 lbs
Resistance : 467 ohms            Activity level : Moderate
Reactance : 51 ohms              Step Test : N/A
--------------------------------------------------------------
           Your Body Composition Results are as follows:


                    TOTAL BODY WATER

Your total body water is 48 liters or 56 %.  The average total body water
for a male is 60 %.  The amount of water in your body is determined by the
amount of lean and fat tissue.  Lean tissue is approximately 71 - 75% water,
while fat tissue is about 14 - 22% water.


                    LEAN BODY MASS

Your lean body weight is 148 pounds or 78 %.  This corresponds to a lean
weight to fat weight ratio of  3.5.  A value of  5.7 or higher is desirable
for you.


                       BODY FAT

Your body fat is  42 pounds or 22 %.  Your body fat should be 12 to 18 %.
Your body fat is  16 pounds above the average for a male of your age and
lean weight.


                INITIAL WEIGHT RECOMMENDATIONS

          Your initial target weight is 170 to 178 pounds
It is suggested that you decrease your weight by at least  16 lbs.  Weight
loss usually includes both fat and lean tissue.  The loss of lean tissue will
be minimized by exercising at least  3 days per week.


                CALORIC RECOMMENDATIONS

Your estimated basal metabolism is 2045 Kcal, based on your age, sex and
lean body mass.  Your estimated total daily caloric requirement is 2556 Kcal,
based on your basal metabolism and activity level.  Calories expended during
exercise should be added to your daily caloric requirements.

A daily caloric intake of 1306 Kcal plus calories expended during exercise
will result in a weight loss of approximately 2.5 lbs/week.

With this dietary/exercise program, it will be possible to increase your
lean to fat ratio and reach your goal weight of 174 lbs in  45 days.
To measure your progress, monitor your Body Composition regularly.
```

Figure 3.11. Body composition profile (sides 1 and 2). This chart, provided by RJL Systems Inc., is the result of a computerized body composition analysis performed on the company's BIA-101 system.

2. Forms the standard for most other methods of body composition analysis.

2. Time consuming.
3. Potentially uncomfortable for the patient.

Method 2: Neutron Activation

Various elements are measured; body fat can be calculated:

Advantages

1. More information can be gained than through any other method.

Disadvantages

1. High cost.
2. Skilled operators needed.
3. Ionizing radiation must be used.

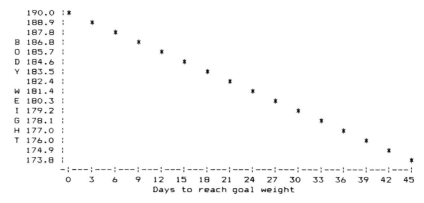

Weight loss for James Michaels

```
        190.0 :*
        188.9 :     *
        187.8 :         *
  B  186.8 :              *
  O  185.7 :                  *
  D  184.6 :                      *
  Y  183.5 :                          *
        182.4 :                              *
  W  181.4 :                                  *
  E  180.3 :                                      *
  I  179.2 :                                          *
  G  178.1 :                                              *
  H  177.0 :                                                  *
  T  176.0 :                                                      *
        174.9 :                                                          *
        173.8 :                                                              *
        -:---:---:---:---:---:---:---:---:---:---:---:---:---:---:---:
          0   3   6   9  12  15  18  21  24  27  30  33  36  39  42  45
                        Days to reach goal weight
```

EXERCISE RECOMMENDATIONS

Aerobic exercises should be done at least 3 days per week,
a minimum of 20 min per session, and at a minimum intensity level of 60 to 80
percent of your maximum heart rate. In your case, your training heart rate zone
is <u>115 to 154</u> beats per min. Regular exercise will promote optimal body
composition (proportionate fat and lean mass).

	TIME IN MINUTES								
EXERCISE	10	20	30	40	50	60	80	90	120
	(Calories expended based on your weight)								
Walking (15-17 min/mile)	69	138	207	276	345	414	551	620	827
Jogging (10-12 min/mile)	141	283	424	565	707	848	1131	1272	1696
Running (9 min/mile)	166	333	499	665	832	998	1330	1497	1996
Swimming (breast stroke)	140	279	419	558	698	838	1117	1256	1675
Cycling (9.4 m.p.h.)	86	172	259	345	431	517	689	776	1034
Racquetball	151	302	452	603	754	905	1206	1357	1810
Squash	183	365	548	731	913	1096	1461	1644	2192
Basketball	119	238	357	476	595	713	951	1070	1427
Football	114	227	341	455	569	682	910	1024	1365
Soccer	115	231	346	462	577	693	924	1039	1386

Figure 3.11 continued.

Method 3: Bioelectric Impedance

Full body composition profile can be obtained:

Advantages

1. Provides rapid analysis of body water, lean body mass, and body fat.
2. Highly accurate.
3. Can be utilized in various physical settings.
4. Safe and comfortable for the patient.

Disadvantages

1. A lack of reliable literature is available.
2. Costly system, but much less so than Method 2.
3. Some standardized tables may underestimate percentage of fat in the obese and overestimate it in the elderly and the very lean.
4. Accuracy of analysis is affected by the presence of certain physical conditions.

Suggested Readings

Anderson MA. Use of height-arm measurement for nutritional selectivity in Sri Lanka school feeding. Am J Clin Nutr 1975;28:775.

Anonymous. Practical clinical assessment of body composition. Nutrition & the M.D. 1988;8:1–2.

Burgert SL, Anderson CF. A comparison of triceps skinfold values as measured by the plastic McGaw caliper and the Lange caliper. Am J Clin Nutr 1970;32:1531–1533.

Cambridge Scientific Industries. The skinfold test: a clinical method in the management of obesity. Cambridge, Maryland, 1975.

Collins JP, McCarthy ID. Assessment of protein nutrition in surgical patients—the value of anthropometrics. Am J Clin Nutr 1979;32:1527–1530.

Dugdale AE. An age-independent anthropometric index of nutritional status. Am J Clin Nutr 1971:24:174.

el Lozy M. The assessment of nutritional state by composite anthropometric measurements. J Trop Pediatr Environ Child Health 1972; 18:3.

Faintuch JL, Faintuch JJ. Anthropometric assessment of nutritional depletion after surgical injury. J Parent and Ent Nutr 1979; (3)5:369–372.

Fletcher RF. The measurement of total body fat with skinfold calipers. Clin Sci 1962;22:333.

Frisancho AR. Triceps skinfold and upper arm muscle size norms for assessment of nutritional status. Am J Clin Nutr 1974;27:1052–58.

Gurney J, Jelliffe D. Arm anthropometry in nutritional assessment; nomogram for rapid calculation of muscle circumference and cross-sectional muscle and fat areas. Am J Clin Nutr 1973:26:912–15.

Jelliffe ER, Jelliffe DB. The arm circumference as a public health index of protein-calorie malnutrition of early childhood. J Trop Pediatr 1969;15:176.

Kanawati AA, McLaren SS. Assessment of marginal malnutrition. Nature (Lond) 1970;228:573.

Krause MV, Mahan LK. Food, nutrition, and diet therapy: a textbook of nutritional care. 7th ed. Philadelphia: WB Saunders, 1984.

Latanick MR, Gallagher-Allred CR. Appraisal of nutritional status. Columbus, Ohio: Department of Family Medicine, The Ohio State University, 1980.

Lukaski HC. Methods of assessment of human body composition: traditional and new. Am J Clin Nutr 1987;46:537–556.

Margo G. Assessing malnutrition with the mid-arm circumference. Am J Clin Nutr 1977;30:835–837.

Martorell R. Upper arm anthropometric indicators of nutritional status. Am J Clin Nutr 1976;29:46.

McArdle WD, Katch FI, Katch VL. Exercise physiology: energy, nutrition, and human performance. 2nd ed. Philadelphia: Lea & Febiger, 1986.

Pearlman P, Hunter G, Hendricks C, O'Sullivan P. Comparison of hydrostatic weighing and bioelectric impedance measurements in determining body compostion pre- and postdehydration. J Orthop Sports Phys Ther 1989;11:451–455.

Rao KV, Singh D. An evaluation of the relationship between nutritional status and anthropometric measurements. Am J Clin Nutr 1970;23:83.

Shils ME, Young VR. (eds) Modern nutrition in health disease. 7th ed. Philadelphia: Lea & Febiger, 1988.

Taber LA, Cook RA. Dietary and anthropometric assessment of adult omnivores, fish-eaters and lacto-ovo-vegetarians. J Am Diet Assoc 1980;76(1):21–29.

Trowbridge FL. Clinical and biochemical characteristics associated with anthropometric nutritional categories. Am J Clin Nutr 1979;32:758–766.

Trowbridge FL, Staehling N. Sensitivity and specificity of arm circumference indicators in identifying malnourished children. Am J Clin Nutr 1980;33:687–696.

Young GA, Hill GL. Assessment of protein-calorie malnutrition in surgical patients from plasma proteins and anthropometric measurements. Am J Clin Nutr 1978;31:429–435.

Zerfas A. The insertion tape: a new circumference tape for use in nutritional assessment. Am J Clin Nutr 1975;28:782–787.

4

Clinical Laboratory Evaluation

The clinical laboratory provides an important mode of nutritional assessment to augment the clinical evaluation. It has been stated that biochemical measurements serve as the most objective method of assessment of the nutritional status of an individual (1). This is due to the fact that they are independent of subjective factors that influence both the examiner and the patient. Brin suggests that biochemical assessment also enables the investigator to detect marginal or preclinical nutrient deficiency states before they manifest themselves clinically or pathologically (2).

Such laboratory assessments usually utilize samples of the patient's body fluids, blood, and urine. When deciding which tests are to be ordered, the practioner must consider several related factors. These include the ultimate purpose of each test and the possibility that other causes are responsible for abnormalities that appear at first to be nutrition related. In addition, the clinician must know the normal values for the laboratory that is being used (see Table 4.1).

Most laboratory tests used in the assessment of nutritional status measure a variety of factors that are of extreme interest to the clinician. Once these tests are conducted, concentrations of essential nutrients can be studied to determine the various causes for any condition that may be present. The practitioner always should remember, however, that such tests—by themselves — will never reveal specific cause of these concentrations; this only can be accomplished through the types of inclusive clinical examinations and case histories discussed elsewhere in this book.

In addition, it must be noted that not all laboratory tests should be given equal weight, nor are all of them equally sensitive to the various factors that they measure (see Table 4.2). Nonetheless, laboratory evaluations do offer the practitioner a wealth of information that cannot be otherwise obtained, and thus they often may prove invaluable in the overall assessment of any patient's nutritional status.

Stages of Development of Nutrient Deficiency

In combination with a laboratory evaluation that the clinician may order, an understanding of the five stages of nutrient deficiency development will be helpful. These stages are:

1. The Preliminary Stage, which is characterized by an inadequate availability of a nutrient due to diet, malabsorption, and/or abnormal metabolism.

Table 4.1
Sample Laboratory Values
Listed here are estimated and sample laboratory values for normal serum, blood cell, normal urine, stool and other specific tests. (From Pemberton C, Gastineau G, eds. Mayo Clinic Diet Manual. Philadelphia: WB Saunders, 1981; Medical Associates Laboratories, Pittsburg, PA.)

Normal serum values

Coagulation Tests: Bleeding time = 1–3 minutes/Ivy; 2–4 minutes Duke
 Coagulation time = 6–10 minutes
 Erythrocyte Sedimentation Rates = 0–10 mm/hour (males); 0–15 mm/hour (females)
 Prothrombin time = 11–16 second control; 70–110% of control value
Amylase = 60–180 Somogyi units/dl
Bilirubin, total = 0.15–1.0 mg/dl
Calcium = 8.5–10.5 mg/dl
Carotene = 48–200 µg/dl
Ceruloplasmin = 27–37 mg/dl
Chloride = 96–108 mEq/liter
CO_2 = 24–32 mEq/liter
Copper = 70–155 µg/dl
Creatinine = 0.7–1.4 mg/dl
Glycohemoglobin = 5.5–8.5%
Glucose, fasting = 65–110 mg/dl
Lipase = under 1.5 units
Lipids
 Total serum = 450–850 mg/dl
 Cholesterol = 120–210 mg/dl (20–30% HDL, 60–70% LDL)
 Triglycerides = 10–190 mg/dl
 Total fatty acids = 190–240 mg/dl
 Phospholipids = 60–350 mg/dl
Magnesium = 1.5–2.5 mEg/liter or 1.8–3 mg/dl
Nitrogen balance = goal of 1–4g/24 hrs. (UUN)
Nitrogen, nonprotein, serum = 15–35 mg/dl
Osmolality, serum = 285–295 mOsm/liter
Oxygen, blood capacity = 16–24 volume % (varies with Hgb)
pH, arterial, plasma = 7.35–7.45
Phenylalanine, serum = less than 3 mg/dl
Phosphatase, serum
 Acid = 0.5–2 Bodansky units
 Alkaline = 2–4.5 Bodansky units (30–135 u/liter)
Phosphate, inorganic, serum = 3–4.5 mg/dl
Phosphorus = 2.5–4 mg/dl
Potassium, serum –3.5–5.5 mEq/liter
Proteins, serum
 Total = 6–8 g/dl
 Albumin = 3.5–5.5 g/dl (45–55% total)
 Globulin = 1.5–3 g/dl
 Prealbumin = 10–40 mg/dl
 Retinol-binding protein = 37.2 µg/dl
 Transferrin = 200–400 mg/dl
Sodium, serum = 136–145 mEq/liter
Sulfates, serum, inorganic = 0.5–1.5 mg/dl
Transaminases (liver, muscle, brain)
 SGOT (AST) = 5–40 units/ml
 SGPT (ALT) = 5–35 units/ml
Urea nitrogen (BUN) = 10–20 mg/dl
Uric acid = 4.0–9.0 mg/dl

Table 4.1 (continued)

Vitamin A = 125–150 IU/dl or 20–80 µg/dl
Vitamin B_6 = 3.6–18.0 µg/liter
Vitamin B_{12} = 200–900 ng/liter
Vitamin C = 0.6–2 mg/dl
Zinc = 0.75–1.4 µg/ml or up to 70 mg/dl
CPK = 0–145 units/liter
LDH = 200–680 units/ml
Erythrocyte count = 4.5–6.2 million/mm³ (males)
                  = 4.2–5.4 million/mm³ (females)
Ferritin = 20–300 ng/ml (males); 20–120 ng/ml (females)
Folate = 2–20 ng/ml
Iron = 75–175 µg/dl (males); 65–165 µg/dl (females)
Iron-binding capacity, total = 240–450 µg/dl (18–59% saturation)
Hematocrit = 40–54% (males); 37–47% (females)
Hemoglobin = 14–17 g/dl (males); 12–15 g/dl (females)
Mean cell volume (MCV) = 80–94 cu/microns
Mean cell hemoglobin (MCH) = 26–32 picograms
Mean cell hemoglobin concentration = 32–36%
White blood cells = 4.8–11.8 thousand/mm³
Lymphocytes = 24–44% total WBC's
TLC = % lymphocytes × WBC/100; normal = >2000/mm³ deficient = <900/mm³

Normal urine values

Acetone = 0
Aldosterone = 6–16 µg/24 hrs
Ammonia = 20–70 mEq/liter
Amylase = 260–950 Somogyi units/24 hrs
Calcium, normal diet = less than 250 mg/24 hrs
Creatine = less than 100 mg/24 hrs (higher in pregnancy, in children)
Creatinine = 15–25 mg/kg BW in 24 hrs
Estrogens = 4–25 µg/24 hrs (males); 4–60 µg/24 hrs (females); (higher in PG)
Hemoglobin, myoglobin = 0
5-hydroxyindoleacetic acid (5-HIAA) = 0
Osmolality = 300–800 mOsm/kg
Oxalate = 20–60 mg/24 hrs
pH = 4.6–8 with average of 6 (diet dependent)
Protein = less than 30 mg/24 hrs (0 qualitative)
Specific gravity = 1.003–1.030
Sugar = 0
Vanillylmandelic Acid (VMA) = 1.8–8.4 mg/24 hrs

Stool values

Fat = less than 7 g/24 hrs in a 3-day period
Nitrogen = less than 2.5 g/day

Other specific tests

Renal Values: GFR = 110–150 ml/min (males); 105–132 ml/min (females)
              Urea Clearance = 40–65 ml/min standard; 60–100 ml/min maximum
Thyroid Values: T_3 (concentration) = 50–210 ng/dl serum
              T_4 (concentration) = 4.8–13.2 µg/dl serum
              TSH = less than or equal to 0.2 micro-U/liter
              Radioactive Iodine Uptake = 9–19% in one hr; 10–50% in 24 hrs
              Protein-bound iodine = 3.6–8.8 µg/dl

Table 4.2
Biochemical Measurements of Nutritional Status[a]
Using this table, the clinician can determine sensitivities by specific nutrients. (From Kraus MV, Mahan LK. Food, nutrition, and diet therapy: a textbook of nutritional care. 7th ed. Philadelphia: WB Saunders, 1984.)

Nutrient	More Sensitive	Less Sensitive
Protein	Plasma amino acids	Total serum protein
	Serum thyroxine-binding pre-albumin	Serum albumin
	Urinary creatinine: height index	
	Urinary hydroxyproline	
	Serum retinol-binding protein	
	Serum transferrin	
Lipids	Serum cholesterol—HDL and LDL	
	Serum triglycerides	
	Lipoproteins	
Vitamin A	Serum carotene	Blood leukocytes
	Serum retinol	
	Liver retinol stores	
	Serum retinol-binding protein	
Vitamin D	Serum 250HD$_3$	Urinary calcium
	Serum 1,25(OH)$_2$D$_3$	Serum phosphorus
	Serum alkaline phosphatase	Serum parathormone
		Serum calcium
Vitamin E	Hydrogen peroxide erythrocyte hemolysis test	Platelet assessment
	Serum or plasma vitamin E	
	Erythrocyte vitamin E	
Vitamin K	Plasma clotting factors II, VII, IX, X	Prothrombin time
Thiamin	Erythrocyte transketolase activity	Blood pyruvate
	Thiamin pyrophosphate effect (TPPE)	Urinary thiamin
Riboflavin	Plasma riboflavin	Urinary riboflavin
	Erythrocyte glutathione reductase	
	Erythrocyte riboflavin	
Nicotinic acid	Urinary N^1-methylnicotinamide	Urinary 2-pyridone
	Urinary 2-pyricone/N-methylnicotinamide	
	Erythrocyte nicotinamide mononucleotide	

2. The Biochemical Stage, which develops when biochemical defects become apparent due to depressed enzyme-coenzyme activity and reduced body fluid levels of a nutrient.
3. The Physiological Stage, which is marked by personality changes and unspecific clinical manifestations of weight loss, lack of appetite, insomnia, and general malaise.
4. The Clinical Stage, which develops with the full clinical appearance of deficiency syndromes.
5. The Pathological Stage, which can be noted by the establishment of specific deficiency disease with specific tissue pathology.

If the levels of an essential nutrient fall below what is required for optimal functioning, a biochemical derangement can occur at the site of cellular activity where the nutrient is required. Thus, impairment of enzymatic function and production of increased quantities of normal metabolites or production of abnormal metabolites can occur.

New knowledge and understanding of the intricate steps in intermediary metabolism, the interrelationship of metabolic pathways, the availability of new analytical instrumentation, and the development of new analytical techniques

Table 4.2 (continued)

Vitamin B_6	Tryptophan load test (mg. xanthurenic and kynurenic acids excreted in urine are measured after tryptophan load) Plasma and erythrocyte pyridoxal phosphate Erythrocyte transaminase-SGOT and SGPT	Urinary pyridoxine excretion (µg/gm. creatinine)
Folic Acid[b]	Red cell folate	Serum folate Bone marrow film Urinary FIGLU excretion Mean corpuscular volume (MCV)
Vitamin B_{12}	Serum B_{12} Erythrocyte B_{12} Serum thimidylate synthetase Urinary methylmalonic acid[b]	Bone marrow film Thin blood film Schilling test
Pantothemic Acid	Blood pantothenic acid	Urinary pantothenic acid
Biotin	Serum biotin	Urinary biotin
Vitamin C	Serum ascorbic acid Leukocyte ascorbic acid Vitamin C saturation	Urinary ascorbic acid
Iron	Iron deposits in bone marrow % saturation of transferin Serum ferritin Protoporphyrin heme	Mean corpuscular volume (MCV) Hemoglobin Hematocrit Thin blood film Serum iron Mean corpuscular hemoglobin concentration (MCHC)
Iodine	Serum protein-bound iodine (PBI) Radioiodine uptake	Urinary iodine Tests for thyroid function
Calcium	Serum alkaline phosphatase	
Phosphorous		Serum phosphorus
Zinc	Serum and plasma zinc	Hair zinc
Magnesium	Serum magnesium	Urinary magnesium
Copper	Serum copper	

[a]Tests of folate status do not distinguish between folate and B_{12} deficiency except in the case of urine methylmalonic acid, which will distinguish between the two.

all provide for the biochemical assessment of nutriture. Therefore, such laboratory tests will reveal critical information for the practitioner in the following areas:

- Measurement of the circulating nutrient or its metabolite in blood.
- Measurement of the urinary excretion rate of the nutrient or its metabolite.
- Measurement of abnormal metabolic products in blood or urine, resulting from deficient or submarginal intake of nutrients.
- Measurement of changes in blood components or enzyme activities.
- Load, saturation, and isotopic tests.

Utility of Nutrient Information from Biochemical Assays

Use	*Assay*
1. Index of nutrient intake and adequate nutrient absorption.	1. Circulating nutrient in blood or urine.
2. Index of nutrient utilization or metabolic aberration due to nutritional fault.	2. Abnormal or normal metabolites in blood or urine.
3. Index of nutrient utilization as enzyme cofactors.	3. Enzyme activity in selected body fluids.

4. Index of metabolic adaptation in the presence of nutritional deprivation.

5. Therapeutic trial to differentiate between deficiency syndromes and inadequate biochemical utilization of the nutrient.

4. Hormone activity in selected body fluids.

5. Load and saturation tests.

The ability to assess the nutritional status of an individual will improve as the knowledge of metabolic actions and interrelations of individual nutrients at the cellular level grows to produce more efficient and effective functional biochemical assays.

Patient Preparation

Before laboratory testing is initiated, the clinician should be aware that several preanalytical factors may have an impact on the process. These include diet, as well as any medications or nutritional supplements that the patient might be using. Each of these are discussed below.

Effect of Diet on Laboratory Testing

One of the major factors that may affect laboratory values is the diet of a patient before testing. An understanding and awareness of dietary effects can contribute greatly to accurate test interpretation.

Because prior diet can cause changes in various analytes, it generally is stated that patients should be in a fasting state before a planned specimen collection. However, it must be noted that prolonged fasting (more than 24 hours of total fasting) also can lead to unexpected laboratory results. Healthy persons fasting for 48 hours show the following increases: serum total bilirubin (240%), plasma triglycerides (20%), plasma glycerol (70%), and nonesterified fatty acids (140%); increases in various amino acids in plasma—such as valine, leucine, and isoleucine—also are noted. No change appears in serum cholesterol values (3). In fasting, the activity of adipose tissue hormone-sensitive triglyceride lipase increases, with resulting increases in nonesterified fatty acids and glycerol, the products of triglycerides. Plasma triglyceride rises are attributable to increased incorporation of fatty acids into the glycerol molecule. Increased serum total bilirubin may relate to rises in plasma nonesterified fatty acids (4).

Additionally, 48-hour fasts lead to: a 50% increase in plasma glucagon, a 105% increase in plasma secretin, and a 15% increase in plasma insulin. Ketone bodies (acetone, acetoacetate, and beta-hydroxy-butyrate) increase in both urine and serum. Prolonged fasting may effect dramatic decreases in plasma glucose, most pronounced in women, who may experience values as low as 2.5 mmol/L.

Clinicians aiming to assess the nutritional or hormonal status of patients should obviously instruct the patient to avoid prolonged fasting.

Some foods or nutrients also affect certain laboratory measurements. Meals high in fat increase the value of serum alkaline phosphatase because greater amounts of the intestinal alkaline phosphatase isoenzyme are present. Peak increases occurring 2 hours after the meal are most pronounced in O and B blood types and in Lewis positive secretors. Caffeine causes increased plasma catecholamines, which in turn raises plasma nonesterified fatty acids. Diets high in saturated fatty acids result in increased plasma cholesterol. Those high in protein raise serum values for urea, ammonia, and urate (uric acid). Serum creatinine is not significancly affected by changes in dietary protein and may, therefore, be more reliable than urea in assessing kidney status. Purine-rich diets are associated with increased serum urates.

General physiological effects of eating a meal include increases in serum bile acids, insulin, triglycerides, and glucose, and decreases in serum cortisol, glucagon, catecholamines, and nonesterified fatty acids (5). Thus, the ingestion of a meal (within 6 to 10 hours) also causes changes in various hormones, nutrients, and other hormone-related constituents. Certain stress or tolerance tests exploit such effects; these include glucose tolerance tests, food bile acid stress tests, and various tests of gastrointestinal hormones.

A patient's diet also can influence test results through its effects on methodology. Increased serum turbidity after a meal causes falsely elevated (or possibly depressed) values for analytes measured by absorbency of a test solution at a wavelength where the turbid specimen similarly absorbs light.

There are, however, common laboratory tests used in nutritional assessment that require the patient to be fasting. These include:

Serum albumin
Serum alkaline phosphatase
Serum amylase
Serum urea nitrogen
Total cholesterol
High-density lipoprotein (HDL) cholesterol
Fasting glucose
Lipoprotein electrophoresis
Serum phosphorus
Serum aspartate aminotransferase (AST)
Serum alanine aminotransferase (ALT)
Serum gamma glutamyltranspeptidase (GGT)
Serum protein electrophoresis
Serum total protein
Serum triglycerides
Serum uric acid
Serum/plasma zinc
Serum/plasma vitamin A

Effect of Medication and Nutritional Supplements on Laboratory Testing

Drugs, including vitamin and mineral supplements, also may affect laboratory test results. This can occur by three basic mechanisms. They can cause physiological changes in the concentrations of test substances (i.e., increased ceruloplasmin by birth control pills), have a toxic effect on tissues and organs (i.e., increased liver enzymes by steroids), and cause chemical and physical interference (i.e., increased uric acid by vitamin C).

A variety of vitamin and mineral supplements can have a decided impact (inc. = increase; dec. = decrease) on laboratory test values. These include:

Vitamin A
  Serum bilirubin   Inc.
  Serum cholesterol   Inc.
  Serum vitamin A   Inc.
  Blood hemoglobin   Dec.
  Blood hematocrit   Dec.
  Blood red cell count   Dec.
  Blood white cell count   Dec.
  Blood sedimentation rate   Inc.
Vitamin D

Serum alkaline phosphatase	Inc.
Serum calcium	Inc.
Serum cholesterol	Inc.
Serum creatinine	Inc.
Serum phosphate	Inc.
Serum urea nitrogen	Inc.
Urine calcium	Inc.
Urine phosphate	Inc.
Urine protein	Inc.
Serum vitamin D	Inc.
Vitamin C	
Serum bilirubin	Inc.
Serum cholesterol	Dec.
Serum creatinine	Inc.
Serum glucose	Inc.
Serum lactic dehydrogenase	Dec.
Serum aspartate aminotransferase (AST)	Inc.
Serum triglyceride	Dec.
Serum uric acid	Inc.
Urine glucose	Dec.
Urine hemoglobin	Dec.
Urine urobilinogen	Dec.
Urine—uric acid	Inc.
Plasma/serum vitamin C	Inc.
Urine vitamin C	Inc.
Vitamin E	
Urine porphobilinogen	Dec.
Urine uroporphyrin	Dec.
Plasma/serum and tocopherol	Inc.
Nicotinic acid	
Serum alkaline phosphatase	Inc.
Plasma insulin	Inc.
Serum beta-lipoproteins	Dec.
Serum bilirubin	Inc.
Serum cholesterol	Dec.
Serum glucose	Inc.
Serum aspartate aminotransferase (AST) Inc.	
Serum triglycerides	Dec.
Serum uric acid	Inc.
Urine glucose	Inc.
Urine uric acid	Dec.
Urine ketones	Inc.
Urine bilirubin	Inc.
Iron salts	
Serum iron	Inc.
Serum alanine aminotransferase (ALT)	Inc.
Serum total iron binding capacity	Inc.
Urine protein	Inc.
Calcium	
Serum calcium	Inc.
Serum magnesium	Dec.
Urine calcium	Inc.
Urine magnesium	Dec.
Phosphates	

Serum calcium	Dec.
Plasma parathyroid hormone	Inc.
Serum phosphate	Inc.
Serum alkaline phosphatase	Dec.
Serum total acid phosphatase	Dec.
Serum potassium	Dec.
Urine calcium	Dec.
Urine magnesium	Dec.
Urine phosphate	Inc.
Magnesium	
Serum alkaline phosphatase	Inc.
Serum calcium	Dec.
Serum magnesium	Inc.
Copper	
Serum ceruloplasmin	Inc.
Serum copper	Inc.
Serum sodium	Inc.
Serum total acid phosphatase	Dec.
Serum bilirubin	Dec.
Serum calcium	Inc.
Serum lactic dehydrogenase	Inc.
Serum SGOT (AST)	Inc.
Serum SGPT (ALT)	Inc.
Zinc	
Serum alkaline phosphatase	Dec.

Clinical Implications of Common Laboratory Tests

The relationship between nearly two dozen elements on a patient's nutritional status may be revealed in the laboratory. The role of these various elements, as well as the implications of each in an assessment of the patient, are discussed below.

Serum Alkaline Phosphatase

This is a general name given to a group of phosphatases that display maximal activity in the range pH 9.0 to 10.5. They are widely distributed in the liver, bone, placenta, and intestine. Their precise biochemical role is unknown, but it appears to be related to cell membrane transport.

Increased In:

Vitamin D deficiency
Celiac sprue disease
Osteomalacia/rickets
Alcoholism
Hypermetabolic osteopenia
Vitamin K therapy
Third trimester of pregnancy
Recent ingestion of fatty meal
Children—normal bone growth
Osteoblastic bone disease
  Paget's disease
  Hyperparathyroidism

Primary and metastatic tumors
Osteogenesis imperfecta
Healing fracture
Polyostotic fibrous dysplasia
Cushing syndrome
Marble bone disease
Hyperphosphatasia
Market hyperthyroidism
Liver disease—obstruction and cholestasis
   Nodules in the liver (tumor, abscess, etc.)
   Biliary duct obstruction
Adverse reaction to therapeutic drug

Decreased In:

Vitamin C deficiency
Protein malnutrition
Hypervitaminosis D
Vitamin B$_{12}$ deficiency
Folic acid deficiency
Magnesium deficiency
Milk-alkali syndrome
Lactosuria
Hypophosphatasia
Zinc deficiency
Chondrodystrophy
Whipple's disease
Hypothyroidism
Hypoparathyroidism
Zollinger-Ellison syndrome
Collection of blood in EDTA, fluoride, or oxalate

Serum Alanine Aminotransferase (ALT)

This enzyme, still frequently called serum glutamic pyruvic transaminase (SGPT), is found almost exclusively in the soluble fraction of the cell and in high concentration only in the hepatocyte.

Increased In:

Viral hepatitis
Infectious mononucleosis
Malignant neoplasm of liver
Alcoholism
Drug dependence
Muscular dystrophy
Acute myocardial infarction
Cirrhosis
Cholangitis
Shock
Heat stroke
Heavy metal toxicity
Crush injury
Dermatomyositis/Polymyositis

Decreased In:

Exercise
Thiamine deficiency

Serum Albumin

This protein is synthesized in the parenchymal cells of the liver and has a relatively long plasma half-life of 2 to 3 weeks. It mostly is responsible for maintaining the colloid ancotic pressure of plasma and acting as a nonspecific transport mechanism for a number of substances, including fatty acids, urate, calcium, bilirubin, and various drugs.

Increased In:

Dehydration
Recent exercise
Lipemic or turbid serum

Decreased In:

Protein malnutrition
Malabsorption
Celiac sprue disease
Vitamin C deficiency
Whipple's disease
Nephrotic syndrome
Lactosuria
Liver diseae
Stress (surgery, burns, injury)
Ulcerative colitis
Collagen diseases
Analbuminemia
Protein-losing enteropathy
Malignancy
Chronic infection
Alcohol
Hyperthyroidism
Diabetes mellitus
Pancreatitis
Myocardial infarction

Serum Aspartate Aminotransferase (AST)

This enzyme still is known widely as serum glutamic oxaloacetic transaminase (SGOT). It is present in most tissues but is noted especially in skeletal and cardiac muscle, liver, and kidney. There are two major isoenzymes, one cytoplasmic and the other mitochondrial. Although both isoenzymes have been demonstrated in plasma after tissue damage, their differentiation has not been shown to be of much diagnostic value.

Increased In:

Myocardial infarction
Acute rheumatic carditis
Cardiac surgery

Recent angiocardiography
Recent external cardiac massage
Hepatitis
Malignant infiltration of liver
Cholangitis
Infectious mononucleosis
Alcohol ingestion
Pulmonary infarction
Salicylates
Acute pancreatitis
Trauma—surgery, crush injury
Carbon monoxide poisoning
Heat stroke
After intramuscular injection
Muscular dystrophy
Dermatomyositis
Myoglobinuria
Acute attack of gout
Hypothyroid myopathy
Cirrhosis
Recent intensive exercise
Cerebral infarction
Hemolysis

Decreased In:

Thiamine deficiency
Pregnancy
Abnormal pyridoxol metabolism
Severe liver disease
Chronic hemodialysis
Uremia
Diabetic ketoacidosis

Serum Amylase

This enzyme is secreted into the duodenum where it participates in the hydrolysis of macromolecular carbohydrates such as starch and glycogen. The principal application of amylase determinations is in the evaluation of exocrine pancreatic function.

Increased In:

Acute pancreatitis
Acute exacerbation of chronic pancreatitis
Perforated peptic ulcer
Postoperative upper abdominal surgery
Obstruction of pancreatic duct
Acute alcohol ingestion
Salivary gland disease
Advanced renal insufficiency
Macroamylasemia
Renal disease
Chronic malabsorption

Decreased In:

Necrotic pancreatitis
Hepatitis
Cholecystitis
Severe burns
Thyrotoxicosis
Toxemia of pregnancy
Poisoning
Adrenocortical stress
Lipemic sample
Protein malnutrition

Serum (Total) Bilirubin

The end product of hemoglobin breakdown, the serum (total) bilirubin, includes both unconjugated and conjugated forms.

Increased In:

Prolonged fasting
Gilbert's disease
Hepatic cellular damage
Biliary duct obstruction
Hemolytic states

Decreased In:

Iron deficiency anemia

Blood Urea Nitrogen (BUN)

Urea is the primary end product of protein metabolism and is excreted almost entirely by the kidneys. Urea nitrogen determinations, along with serum creatinine, serve as useful tests for renal function.

Increased In:

High protein diet
Excessive protein catabolism
  Gastrointestinal bleeding
  Fever
  Sepsis
Congestive heart failure
Salt and water depletion
  Vomiting
  Diarrhea
Diuresis
Urinary tract obstruction
Renal failure

Decreased In:

Severe liver damage
Low protein-high carbohydrate diet
Celiac disease

Nephrotic syndrome
Acromegaly
Infancy
Late pregnancy
Overhydration

Serum Calcium

Serum calcium is an important element in maintaining proper neuromuscular excitability and in the clotting mechanism. Calcium circulates in the blood in three forms. The ionic calcium, which is metabolically active, accounts for about 50% of the circulating calcium. About 5% is complexed to amino acids and other chelating agents, whereas the remainder (45%) is bound to albumin. When interpreting calcium values it is important to take into account the protein status of the patient.

Increased In:

Dehydration
Hypervitaminosis D
Hyperparathyroidism
Lytic bone tumors
Multiple myeloma
Sarcoidosis
Malignancy
Hyperthyroidism
Alcoholism
Hypophosphatasia
Milk-alkali syndrome
Exercise
Thiazide drugs
Venous stasis during collection

Decreased In:

After recent carbohydrate ingestion
Vitamin D deficiency
Steatorrhea
Celiac sprue disease
Lactosuria
Protein malnutrition
Alcoholism
Acute and chronic pancreatitis
Hypoparathyroidism
Whipple's disease
Pseudohypoparathyroidism
Analbuminemia
Renal failure
Nephrotic syndrome

Carbon Dioxide (CO_2)

Carbon dioxide and water are products of oxygen metabolic processes. The main route of elimination of CO_2 is through the lungs. The depth and rapidity of a person's breathing help control blood CO_2 levels. Therefore, the primary purpose of the test is to measure ventilation.

Increased In:

Respiratory acidosis from asthma, emphysema, and severe chest injuries
Metabolic alkalosis due to diuretic drugs, steroid hormones, or antacids
Vomiting
Intestinal obstruction
Starvation
Hyperactive adrenal glands

Decreased In:

Metabolic acidosis caused by drug poisoning
Diarrhea
Liver disease
Kidney disease
Diabetes mellitus
Hyperventilation

Serum Cholesterol

Serum cholesterol is a sterol that is normally found in all body cells and in blood plasma. Cholesterol is obtained from the diet or synthesized in the liver or intestinal mucosa for release in association with lipoproteins.

Increased In:

Recent ingestion of a meal
Hyperlipoproteinemia
Gout
Hypertension
Hypothyroidism
Diabetes mellitus
Arteriosclerosis
Ischemic heart disease
Biliary obstruction
Cirrhosis
Pregnancy
Chronic renal failure
Nephrotic syndrome
Stress

Decreased In:

Starvation
Steatorrhea
Chronic anemia
Celiac sprue disease
Hyperthyroidism
Tangier disease
Hypobvetalipoproteinemia and abetalipoproteinemia
Protein malnutrition
Severe liver cell damage
Cortisone and ACTH therapy
Clofibrate therapy
Estrogen therapy
Large doses of nicotinic acid

Plasma Chloride

Plasma chloride is a major anion in plasma, although little is known about its specific role and regulation. It appears to be present to maintain electroneutrality as a complementary anion with bicarbonate.

Increased In:

Dehydration
Exercise
Hyperparathyroidism
Diarrhea
Vitamin D deficiency
Diabetes insipidus
Adrenal cortical hyperfunction
Renal tubular acidosis
Fistula of stomach and duodenum
Respiratory alkalosis
Steroid therapy
Chronic pyelonephritis

Decreased In:

Low salt diet
Gastrointestinal loss
Diabetes ketosis
Chronic renal failure
Metabolic alkalosis
Mercurial diuretics
Adrenal cortical deficiency
Respiratory acidosis
Acute intermittent porphyria
Water intoxication

Serum Creatinine

A nonprotein nitrogenous waste product of the body, creatinine is excreted almost entirely by the kidney. Determinations serve as a useful test for evaluating renal function.

Increased In:

Ingestion of roast meat
Gigantism
Acromegaly
Renal failure
Uremia
Severe congestive heart failure
Salicylate therapy
Dehydration

Decreased In:

Hepatolenticular degeneration
Pregnancy
Eclampsia

Serum Creatinine Kinase (CK)

This is a magnesium-dependent enzyme formerly known as creatinine phosphotransferase (CPK). It has three principal molecular forms: BB (brain and other nonmuscle tissues), MMK (skeletal muscle,) and MB (cardiac muscle).

Increased In:

Myocardial infarction
Progressive muscular dystrophy
Muscle crush injury
Severe hemophilia
Cerebral vascular accident
Hypothermia
Tetanus
Carbon monoxide poisoning
Hypothyroidism
Chronic alcoholism
Recent intramuscular injection
Exercise
Prostatic cancer
McArdle's syndrome
Malignant hyperpyrexia

Decreased In:

Hereditary spherocytosis
Pregnancy

Serum or Plasma Glucose

This test reflects carbohydrate metabolism homeostasis. Glucose in the plasma amounts to less than 3 gm, and blood sugar levels are an imperfect reflection of physiological extremes between fasting and feeding. They are affected by exercise as well as by the impact of many diseases.

Increased In:

Diabetes mellitus
Strenuous exercise
Strong emotion, e.g., fear
Vitamin B deficiency
Pancreatitis
Cushing's syndrome
Gigantism and acromegaly
After ACTH injections
Shock
Severe burns
Thyrotoxicosis
Pheochromocytoma
Recent adrenalin injection
Central nervous system lesions

Decreased In:

Starvation
Prolonged exercise
Pregnancy and lactation

Functional reactive hypoglycemia
Alimentary hypoglycemia
Hypoglycemia of early adult onset diabetes
Insulin overdosage
Islet cell tumor
Pancreatitis
Glucagon deficiency
Hypothalamic lesions
Adrenal cortical insufficiency
Hypopituitarism
Diffuse severe liver disease
Oral hypoglycemic medications
Von Gierke's disease
Galactosemia
Fructose intolerance

Serum Gammaglutamyl Transferase (GGT)

This enzyme is distributed in many tissues of the body, including the liver, kidney, spleen, and placenta. GGT is present in the endoplasmic reticulum of the hepatocyte where its activity is increased in situations leading to microsomal enzyme induction.

Increased In:

Recent alcohol ingestion
Hepatitis
Cirrhosis
Obstructive jaundice
Liver metastases
Pancreatitis
Nephrosis
Infectious mononucleosis
Regional ileitis
Hypertriglyceridemia
Cardiac failure
Myocardial infarction
Heavy use of barbiturates
Phenytoin sodium

Decreased In:

GGT enzyme deficiency

Serum Lactic Dehydrogenase (LDH)

This zinc-containing enzyme is widely distributed throughout all body tissues where it is present predominantly in the cytosol. By regulating the interconversion of lactate and pyruvate, it exercises a control over the balance between respiration and glycolysis. There are five isoenzymes, each comprising a tetramer of four subunit polypeptide chains.

Increased In:

Hemolysis
Heavy exercise
Pernicious anemia

Folic acid deficiency, anemia
Acute myocardial infarction
Hepatitis
Cardiovascular surgery
Malignant tumors
Diseases of skeletal muscle
Pulmonary embolus and infarction
Renal infarction
Hypothyroid myopathy
Pneumonia

Decreased In:

X-ray irradiation

Serum Magnesium

Magnesium is a mineral that is active in many biochemical processes, especially in enzyme reactions. When patients have symptoms that include weakness, twitching, and irritability, the test is performed.

Increased In:

Recent ingestion of glucose
Recent ingestion of magnesium salts
Renal failure
Acute and subacute necrosis of liver
Hypothyroidism
Leukemia

Decreased In:

Magnesium deprivation
Protein malnutrition
Celiac sprue disease
Malabsorption
Acute alcoholism
Acute myocardial infarction
Nephrotic syndrome
Hepatic failure
Whipple's disease
Hepatitis
Hyperthyroidism
Epilepsy
Regional enteritis or ileitis
Ulcerative colitis

Inorganic Phosphorus

Inorganic phosphorus is inversely related to calcium, and therefore many causes of elevated calcium also are causes of hypophosphatemia. Phosphorus levels are normally elevated in youth and adolescence.

Increased In:

Renal failure (most common cause in a hospital population)
Healing bone fractures
Diabetic ketosis

Hypoparathyroidism
Hypervitaminosis D

Decreased In:

Continuous use of intravenous glucose in a nondiabetic
Negative nitrogen balance
Rickets
Some hepatic disorders
Osteomalacia
Fanconi's syndrome

Potassium

Potassium is a blood electrolyte that maintains the balance of water within the body cells. It is necessary for enzyme reactions as well as for regulation of heart muscle action.

Increased In:

Diabetes mellitus
Carcinoid syndrome
Acute renal failure
Urethritis
Heat stroke

Decreased In:

Bacillary dysentery
Cholera
Whipple's disease
Malignant neoplasms of the large intestine
Diabetes mellitus
Adrenal cortical hyperfunction
Protein malnutrition
Celiac sprue disease
Malabsorption
Cystinosis
Alcoholism
Congestive heart failure
Asthma
Regional enteritis or ileitis
Cirrhosis of liver

Total Protein

The causes of hyperproteinemia actually are the causes of hyperglobulinemia, since hyperalbuminemia generally is not observed.

Causes for hyperproteinemia:

Acute liver disease (cirrhosis)
Acute and chronic infections
Lupus erythematosus
Rheumatoid arthritis
Myocardial infarction

Gamma G-myeloma
Gamma A-myeloma
Waldenström's macroglobulinemia
Parasitic diseases
Gamma D-myeloma
Nephrotic syndrome
Iron deficiency conditions

Causes for hypoproteinemia:

Low total protein values are derived from the same causes as those listed for hypoalbuminemia. Hypoglobulinemia lowers total protein by lowering the globulin rather than lowering albumin or albumin and globulin.

Sodium

Sodium is one of the blood electrolytes and is essential to maintain normal water metabolism and acid-base balance.

Increased In:

Cholera
Lymphosarcoma
Lymphocytic leukemia
Adrenal cortical hyperfunction
Congestive heart failure
Cerebral hemorrhage
Cerebral thrombosis
Hepatic failure
Dehydration
Acromegaly (early sign)
Diabetes mellitus
Hemolysis—any form

Decreased In:

Epidemic typhus
Rocky Mountain spotted fever
Malaria
Multiple myeloma
Hypothyroidism
Severe adrenal cortical hyperfunction
Celiac sprue disease
Malabsorption
Type V hyperlipoproteinemia
Essential benign hypertension
Recent ingestion of antacids
Hypocalcemia
Cirrhosis of the liver
Alcohol

Uric Acid

Uric acid is one of the end products of the body's protein metabolism. Increased values may be due to the presence of disease or the ingestion of foods with a high uric acid content (sweetbreads, liver, kidney, fish roe, sardines, anchovies).

Increased In:

Gout
Hypertension
Hyperlipidemia
Thiazide diuretics
Renal insufficiency
Atherosclerosis
Prolonged fasting and starvation
Malignancy
Lesch-Nyhan syndrome
Lead poisoning
Alcoholism
Depressive neurosis
Sarcoidosis
Cirrhosis of liver
Toxemia of pregnancy
High protein weight reducing diet
Wilson's disease (hepatolenticular degeneration)
Systemic lupus erythematosus
Lupus nephritis (cause of pulmonary emphysema)
Diabetes mellitus

Decreased In:

Fanconi's syndrome
Hodgkin's disease
Folic acid deficiency anemia
Wilson's disease
Uricosuric drugs

Biochemical Assessment of Nutrients: Carbohydrates

The level—and type—of carbohydrate present in the patient is of prime concern to the clinician. Laboratory evaluation of carbohydrates is demonstrated in the measurement of glucose and the consequences of altered carbohydrate metabolism as reflected in urine, serum, plasma and whole blood (see Fig. 4.1).

Urine Glucose

The presence of glucosuria usually indicates diabetes mellitus. It occurs when the blood glucose level exceeds the reabsorption capacity of the renal tubules, i.e., when the glomerular filtration contains more glucose than the tubules are able to reabsorb (renal threshold). A positive urine test for glucose warrants further laboratory investigation as the patient may have one of a group of conditions associated with incomplete glucose resorption at normal serum levels (renal glucosuria). If a urine reduction test (i.e., clinitest) was used, a reducing sugar other than glucose (lactose, fructose, galactose, etc.) may be present in the urine.

Blood Glucose

1. Plasma or serum values are 15% higher than whole blood.
2. Specimen should be collected with sodium fluoride and potassium oxalate (gray top) to prevent glycolysis and stabilize glucose levels 24 to 48 hours.

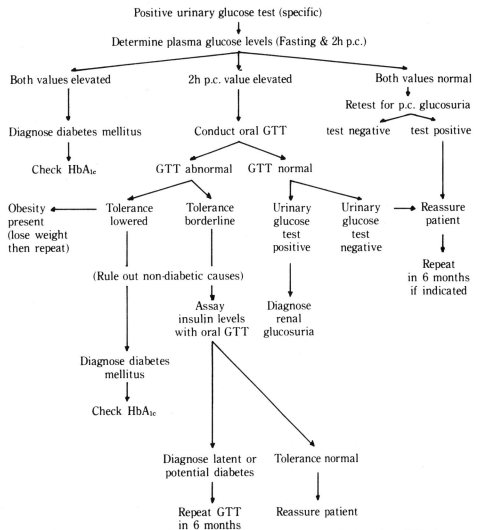

Figure 4.1. Algorithm for investigation of a positive test for glucose in the urine. *GTT*, glucose tolerance test; *HbA1C*, glycosylated hemoglobin; *pc*, postcibal. (Modified from Kellen JA. Applied biochemistry of clinical disorders. New York: Harper & Row, 1980.)

3. Random plasma glucose
   200 mg/dl = diabetes mellitus
4. Fasting plasma glucose
   140 mg/dl = more than one occasion is considered consistent with diagnosis of diabetes mellitus
5. Two-hour postcibal (postprandial) plasma glucose
   110 mg/dl or less = rules out the possibility of diabetes
   110 to 180 mg/dl = equivocal
   180 mg/dl or greater = consistent with diabetes mellitus

Oral Glucose Tolerance Test

An oral glucose tolerance test (OGTT) is not usually required before a diagnosis can be made, and it therefore may be bypassed because of its potential for discomfort to the patient. (Carbohydrates must be added to the patient's diet for 3 days before the test, glucose is introduced according to body weight, and blood is taken at four intervals.) The OGTT still may be called for, however, if the

Table 4.3
Interpretation of the OGTT

There are many formulas and schemes for interpreting the values obtained from an OGTT. Herein are the most popular criteria for diagnosis. All values cited are for plasma samples using a true glucose procedure (reported in milligrams per deciliter, unless otherwise designated).

INTERPRETATION OF THE OGTT

Method	Fasting	1 hr.	1½ hrs.	2 hrs.	3 hrs.	Comments
Fajans and Conn		<185	<160	<140		All three must be abnormal for diagnosis.
USPHS*	<110	<170		<120	<110	
Mosenthal and Barry		<151		<101		
American Diabetes Association (1968)	<115	<185	<165	<140		Elevated fasting or all three abnormal.
Joslin Clinic	<110	<150		<120	<110	

DANOWSKI—Sum of four samples**
at intervals: (A) 0, 30, 60, 120, 180 minutes.

WILKERSON POINT SYSTEM—
two or more points are diagnostic of diabetes.

	Normal	Equivocal	Diabetes	Interval	Fasting	1 hr.	2 hrs.	3 hrs.
A	<575	576-920	921 or more	Value	>130	>195	>140	>130
B	<518	519-805	806 or more	Points	1	½	½	1

*United States Public Health Service   **Autoanalyzer ferricyanide procedure

THE ORAL GLUCOSE TOLERANCE TEST (75 GM. ORAL GLUCOSE):

Diagnosis	Plasma Glucose Level (mg/dl)		
	1 hr.	2 hrs.	3 hrs.
Diabetes Mellitus	200 or	200 or	
Impaired Glucose Tolerance	140-200	200 or	
Gestational Diabetes	190	165	145
"Normal"		140	

practitioner finds it necessary to resolve certain unanswered questions (see Table 4.3). For example, it will help in the determination of the patient's tolerance for an unusually large amount of glucose: a normal body can dispose of it within 2 hours, whereas an abnormal one cannot.

Indications

Indications for OGTT are apparent in clinical situations suggesting the presence of diabetes mellitus, when definite hyperglycemia is absent. These include:

Family history of diabetes
Retinopathy
Periperal vascular disease
Unexplained neuropathy
Furunculosis
Obesity (especially if there is a family history of diabetes)
Birth weight greater than 9 pounds
Presence during pregnancy
History of big babies, fetal or perinatal losses, or congenital anomalies
Glucosuria
Excessive weight gain
Toxemia
Family history of diabetes
Equivocal plasma glucose
Reactive hypoglycemia

Contraindications

OGTT is unnecessary for the diagnosis of diabetes when the following conditions are present:

Consistently elevated fasting glucose levels
Episodes of diabetic ketoacidosis

OGTT is also unnecessary in the presence of "stresses" that may temporarily alter glucose tolerance, such as:

Undernutrition or starvation
Debilitation
Acute febrile illness
Recent myocardial infarction
Recent cerebrovascular accident or head injury
Recent surgery

Patient preparation

- Diet: 150 gm of carbohydrate for 3 days before testing.
- Medication: If affects test, discontinue for 3 days.
- Fasting: No food for at least 8 hours before testing.
- Miscellaneous: Smoking and excessive exercise should be avoided at least 8 hours before testing.
- Postponement: Unexpected illness or food ingestion.

Testing

- Time: Test should be started in morning (7:00 to 9:00 a.m.).
- Glucose load: Follow American Diabetic Association standard (75 gm).
- Patient behavior: Avoid physical exertion, emotional stress, alcohol, and stimulants such as tobacco, coffee, and tea during the test.
- Specimen Collection: Fasting 1, 1 1/2, 2, and 3 hours (extended collection for 5 to 6 hours for reactive hypoglycemia).

Factors affecting oral glucose tolerance test results

Technical:

Glucose load
Route of administration
Time of day and last meal
Type of blood sample
Analytical method for glucose

Host:

Dietary preparation
Level of physical activity
Coexistent endocrinopathies
Administration of drugs
Age

Glycosylated Hemoglobins (HbA1C)

A measure of the body's glycosylated hemoglobin is an indication of its long-term blood glucose level. This gives the practitioner a method of determining long-term blood glucose control: The longer the patient's blood glucose is high, for example, the higher the glycosylated hemoglobin. Because the determination it offers is long-term, however, this measure is not helpful in adjusting daily insulin doses.

In using this measure, the clinician should consider:

- 90 to 95% of adult human hemoglobin is A.
- HbA1 is the sum of minor hemoglobin (10% of total).
- HbA1c is the largest component (4 to 8%).
- As red blood cells (RBCs) circulate during a 120-day span, glucose molecules become attached to hemoglobin (aminoterminal valine of the beta-chain).
- The glycosylation is a slow and nearly irreversible process with the rate of HbA1C formation dependent upon the glucose concentration in the blood.
- HbA1C concentration in diabetes has been shown to correlate with fasting plasma glucose, mean daily plasma glucose, and 24-hour urinary excretion of glucose. It is considered to be a better indicator of long-term control than glucose determinations.

Advantages

1. A quantitative test is not dependent upon patient cooperation.
2. It is independent of time of day.
3. It allows for a simplified follow-up and gives a definitive end point.
4. It examines the relationship between metabolic control and complications.

Limitations

1. It is not helpful in deciding on insulin changes.
2. It does not reflect occurrence of hypoglycemia.
3. It is altered in RBC disorders.
4. HbF (in infants and pregnant women) interferes withmeasurements.

Serum Insulin

Serum insulin assays after oral glucose load distinguish type I (insulin dependent) from type II (insulin independent) diabetes mellitus. Those with induced serum insulin peaks of less than 60 U/ml developed diabetic complications of retinopathy, sensory neuropathy, and renal disease. These individuals have true insulin deficiency (type I).

Suggested Workup for Reactive Hypoglycemia

1. Five-hour oral glucose tolerance test (insulin levels optional).
2. If and when patient develops symptoms during the test, a plasma glucose and cortisol should be drawn at onset of symptoms. Another specimen for plasma cortisol should be obtained 30 minutes later.

In bona fide reactive hypoglycemia, the plasma glucose should fall to a level less than 50 mg/dl during symptoms, and the plasma cortisol exhibits a rise of at least 100 ug/dl to document that the plasma glucose has fallen to a level sufficient to set off counterregulatory mechanisms.

Evaluation of Patient Response

Cause: Functional Hypoglycemia

- Fasting blood sugar—Normal: 60 to mg/dl.
- Initial blood sugar response—Normal during first 2 hours. Maximum below 160 mg/dl. Two-hour level below 110 mg/dl.

- Final blood sugar response—A drop to the lowest level (below 45 mg/dl many times) between second and fourth hours.

Cause: Mild diabetes (Secondary Hypoglycemia)

- Fasting blood sugar—Usually normal; not above 110 mg/dl.
- Initial blood sugar response—Above normal during the first 2 hours; 1-hour level at least 160 mg%; 2-hour level at least 120 mg%.
- Final blood sugar response—A drop to as low as 45 mg/dl between third and fifth hours.

Cause: Postgastroenterostomy Hypoglycemia (Dumping Syndrome)

- Fasting blood sugar—Normal
- Initial blood sugar response—A peak of 200 to 300 mg/dl within 1 hour.
- Final blood sugar response—A drop to as low as 45 mg/dl or lower between second and fourth hours.

Biochemical Assessment of Nutrients: Protein

Next, the clinician may determine the amount of protein present in the patient's body by laboratory analysis. Comparisons and explanations of five possible measurements are provided below.

Total protein (Serum)

Measurement of total serum protein is of little value in determining the protein status of an individual.

Albumin

Serum albumin is a valid measure of nutritional state for epidemiological surveys. Due to the low sensitivity and specificity, however, it is a poor parameter for evaluating the individual patient's nutritional state. Nonetheless, it still may be a prime indicator of protein malnutrition if values are less than 3 gm. And it should be noted that serum albumin may be reduced for reasons other than nutritional deficiency, such as liver disease or gastrointestinal protein loss.

Transferrin (Serum)

Transferrin is an iron transport protein that is produced by the liver and transports iron to the liver and spleen for storage. Because it has a shorter half-life than albumin (7 to 8 days) and a smaller distribution space, transferrin is a sensitive indicator of protein malnutrition. However, it has limited usefulness in the presence of iron deficiency, liver disease, and gastrointestinal disease.

Retinol-binding protein (RBP) (Serum)

Retinol-binding protein is a vitamin A transport protein that has a half-life of 12 hours. It is an early marker of restoration of protein stores.

Prealbumin (PA) (Serum)

This is a thyroid-binding protein that has a half-life of 2 days. It correlates more closely with protein malnutrition than any other hepatic secretory proteins.

Biochemical Assessment of Nutrients: Lipids

Often used interchangeably with "fats," lipids are a heterogeneous group of compounds related to the fatty acids. This includes ordinary fats and oils, waxes, and related compounds. Their significance in the assessment of nutritional status can be determined by a laboratory analysis of two different areas.

Cholesterol

See the prior section in this chapter on "Serum Cholesterol" for complete details.

Triglycerides

Triglycerides comprise the greatest amount (by weight) of lipids in the blood. They come from fats in the diet and also can be manufactured by the liver. Alcohol and carbohydrates, more than fatty foods, cause a great increase in blood triglyceride levels.

Increased In:

Familial hyperlipidemia
Liver diseases
Nephrotic syndrome
Hypothyroidism
Diabetes mellitus (higher values correlate with hyperglycemia and poorer control of diabetes; reduced by insulin therapy)
Alcoholism
Gout
Pancreatitis
Von Gierke's disease
Acute myocardial infarction (rise to peak in 3 weeks; increase may persist for 1 year)

Decreased In:

Congenital abetalipoproteinemia
Malnutrition

Biochemical Assessment of Nutrients: Vitamin, Mineral Status

A laboratory analysis of vitamin and mineral status may help the practitioner greatly in assessing the patient's nutritional condition. An examination of the indications and requirements related to 18 of these elements is provided below.

Vitamin A

Serum carotene
   Limited value
   Indicates recent dietary intake
Serum vitamin A (retinol)
   Only reliable test
   Fasting specimen required
   Reflects vitamin A status and fat malabsorption

Can be decreased in liver disease and infections
Retinol binding protein (RBP)
  Evaluates vitamin A transport system
  Ratio of retinol to RBP is a promising technique

Vitamin D

Serum alkaline phosphatase
  Increased in vitamin D deficiency
Serum calcium and phosphate
  Decreased in rickets and osteomalacia
Vitamin D (serum)
  Radioimmunoassay (RIA) techniques are routinely used today to measure
    vitamin D status, and they can also measure active metabolic form (1,25
    DHCC).

Vitamin E

Alpha tocopherol (serum, RBC)
  Preferred method
  Recently developed gas-liquid chromatographic technique
Erythrocyte hemolysis—H_2O_2
  Indirect measurement
  Incubate RBCs in H_2O_2 for a period of time and measure hemoglobin pro-
    duced by hemolysis.

Vitamin K

Prothrombin Time
Serum K (phylloquinone) and K_2 (menaquinone)
  High pressure liquid chromatography (HPLC), fluorimetry

Vitamin C

Plasma ascorbate
Urinary ascorbate
Leukocyte ascorbate assay
  This measures tissue stores of vitamin C.
Vitamin C loading test
Lingual vitamin C test
  Not specific for C
  Does not reflect tissue stores

Vitamin B₁ (Thiamine)

Blood and urine thiamine
  Screening technique with high pressure liquid chromatography
Blood pyruvic and lactic acid
  Indirect method
  Lack of specificity
  Increased after glucose load and exercise
Red blood cell transketolase
  Biochemical function test
  High sensitivity and specificity

Vitamin B₂ (Riboflavin)

RBC riboflavin
Urine riboflavin
RBC glutathione reductase
  Enzyme activity measured

Niacin

N-methyl nicotinamide (urine)
Serum niacin
  This is measured by high pressure liquid chromatography

Vitamin B₆ (Pyridoxine)

Hypochromic anemia
Urinary 4-pyridoxic acid
Tryptophan loading
  Xanthurenic and kynurenic acid are increased in the urine in deficiency
    states.
B₆ stimulation of enzymes
  SGOT/SGPT
Leukocyte pyridoxal phosphate
  High pressure liquid chromatography

Pantothenic Acid

Blood and urine pantothenic acid
  Microbiological assays using *Lactobacillus plantarum*
  RIA, fluorimetry

Biotin

Blood biotin
  Microbiological assay

Folic Acid

For details, see the full section on Anemias in Chapter 6.

Iron

For details, see the full section on Anemias in Chapter 6.

Vitamin B₁₂

For details, see the full section on Anemias in Chapter 6.

Iodine

Urinary iodine
Plasma iodine—Determined by neutron activation analysis
Routine thyroid tests (for details, see the full section on Thyroid Function Tests
  later in this chapter).

Calcium

Calcium serum
  Serum ionized calcium—serum
  Urine calcium

Magnesium

Serum/urine magnesium

Zinc

Serum/urine zinc
Leukocyte zinc
Serum alkaline phosphatase
  Pretherapeutic and posttherapeutic serum alkaline phosphatase increases
    after zinc therapy.

Liver Function Tests

The liver, the largest glandular organ in the body, also is one of the most critical during the process of food metabolism. It performs the most numerous and most varied functions of all of the body's organs, and the majority of the end products of digestion are transported to it. It plays a major role, therefore, in the laboratory assessment of a patient's nutritional status.

Specifically, liver function (and overall nutritional status) may be altered dramatically by the presence of liver disease. A number of tests, then, are used to answer the following important questions:

Is liver disease present?
What type of disease?
What is the prognosis?

Details on the various methods used to answer each of these questions are offered below.

Presence of Liver Disease

In order to determine by laboratory analysis whether liver disease is present, the clinician should consider the following:

- SGOT (AST) is the preferred indicator of cell necrosis.
- ALP is the preferred indicator of cholestasis.
- BSP is the most sensitive indicator of defective anion metabolism; direct bilirubin is a safe and simple substitute.
- Bile acids are the most sensitive liver function tests.
- GGT (gammaglutamyl transpeptidase or transferase) may be the best indicator of infiltrative liver disease and minimal alcoholic damage.
- Hepatitis-related antigens and antibodies may be required if viral infection is suspected.

Specific Diagnosis of Liver Disease

Once the practitioner has initiated a laboratory analysis and determined that liver disease is present, the following should be considered during the diagnostic stage:

- Marked elevated SGOT favors necrosis due to viral, toxic, or circulatory causes (except for acute alcoholic hepatitis, in which increase may be moderate).
- Marked elevated ALP and cholesterol favor cholestasis.
- Elevated SGOT and gamma globulin favor chronic aggressive hepatitis.
- Beta-gamma bridging on electrophoresis suggests cirrhosis.
- Mild unconjugated hyperbilirubinemia suggests hemolysis or Gilbert's disease.
- Isolated ALP elevation with normal bilirubin may represent bone disease (normal GGT will exclude liver as source).
- Isolated hepatic ADP elevation with normal bilirubin suggests benign infiltrative liver disease or calculus in a hepatic duct.
- Elevated ALP and LDH with normal bilirubin suggest malignant infiltrative disease or congestive heart failure.
- Presence of antimitochondrial antibody with elevated ADP, cholesterol, and IgM suggests primary biliary cirrhosis rather than extrahepatic obstruction.
- Alpha-fetoprotein in a cirrhotic patient using immunodiffusion suggests hepatoma.

Severity of Liver Disease or Prognosis

After the presence of liver disease has been noted and a specific diagnosis is made, a prognosis must be offered.

Poor prognosis is indicated by:

An albumin level less than 3 mg/100 ml.
A total bilirubin greater than 4 mg/100 ml in acute liver failure.
A prothrombin time greater than 4 seconds over control, uncorrectable with vitamin K.
A marked rise in unconjugated bilirubin with little or no failure.
A falling SGOT (AST) level in liver failure.

Good prognosis is indicated by:

A rise in AFP level in acute liver failure.
A rise in albumin with a fall in globulin in chronic aggressive hepatitis.
A fall in SGOT (AST) or ALP with appropriate therapy.
A decrease in AFP with therapy of hepatoma.

Preferred Test Grouping

The preferred test grouping for the simultaneous detection, diagnosis, and assessment of severity of liver disease is:

Alanine aminotransferase (SGPT) (ALT)
Alkaline phosphatase
Total and direct bilirubin
Serum protein electrophoresis

Summary

The clinical situation determines the choice of hepatic function tests. Alkaline phosphatase (ALP) and aspartate aminotransferase (AST) tests serve to detect disease, and when used in combination with gammaglutamyl transpeptidase (LDH), albumin, globulin, and GGT tests they are useful for routine differential diagnosis. Prothrombin time indicates severity of disease. Interpretation is facilitated by attention to ALP or AST predominance; the relationship of LDH, ALP, and bilirubin; and the ratio of GGT to ALP. Abnormalities on routine tests frequently do no more than point out the need for more definitive procedures.

Evaluating Liver Function

To:	Do these tests:
Detect occult liver disease	Bile acids
Distinguish hepatocellular and obstructive jaundice	SGOT (AST) Alkaline phosphatase Prothrombin time SGPT (ALT) Serum protein electrophoresis GGT
Distinguish intrahepatic and extrahepatic obstructive jaundice	SGOT (AST) Serum protein electrophoresis Urinary and fecal urobilinogen Antimitochondrial antibody Biopsy
Detect hepatoma	Alpha-fetoprotein
Detect metastatic carcinoma	Alkaline phosphatase SGOT (AST) SGPT (ALT) Biopsy
Detect cholestasis	Alkaline phosphatase GGT Total bilirubin
Detect hepatocellular involvement	SGOT (AST) SGPT (ALT) LDH LDH isoenzymes
Detect cirrhosis	Total bilirubin SGOT (AST) SGPT (ALT) Alkaline phosphatase Total protein Serum protein electrophoresis Urine bilirubin
Detect chronic passive congestion (CPC) of the liver	Total bilirubin Urine urobilinogen SGOT (AST) SGPT (ALT) LDH LDH isoenzymes Alkaline phosphatase
Detect hepatitis A	SGOT (AST) SGPT (ALT) Ha Ag anti-HAV IgM anti-HAB Total bilirubin

Detect hepatitis B	SGOT (AST)
	SGPT (ALT)
	Total bilirubin
	HBsAg
	HBeAg
	DNA-P
	anti-HBs
	anti-HBe
	anti-HBc
Detect alcoholic hepatitis	STOT (AST)
	SGPT (ALT)
	Alkaline phosphatase
	White blood cell count
	Alcoholic hyaline antigen
	Alcoholic hyaline antibody
Detect alcoholic liver disease "other than hepatitis"	Total bilirubin
	Alkaline phosphatase
	SGOT
	Uric acid
	LDH
	Total protein, albumin
	GGP
	Urine urobilinogen
	Serum magnesium

Thyroid Function Tests

The thyroid gland is an endocrine organ whose hormones have a direct effect on the body's rate of metabolism. The hormones secreted by the thyroid regulate the oxidative rate and, therefore, the rate of heat production and energy liberation of all cells in the body. A multitude of thyroid function tests are now available to aid the clinician in the diagnosis of thyroid disease (see Fig. 4.2).

Despite the plethora of options, however, the practitioner always must remember that the laboratory test requested may not be appropriate and the test results may lead to the wrong diagnosis and treatment. Some of the problems are due to the vast number of available tests, the varied terms used to describe the tests, and the general failure of clinicians to understand exactly what is measured by the requested tests.

Normal and Abnormal Thyroid Function

The thyroid gland secretes several hormones under normal conditions. These include triiodothyronine (or T3), thyroxine (or T4), reverse triiodothyronine (or rT3, which is metabolically inactive), and calcitonin. These hormones all are made from iodine—a dietary nutrient that serves no other function in the human body—and their release is regulated by thytotropin (the thyroid-stimulating hormone, or TSH). Additionally, thyroid hormones have an effect on the metabolism of carbohydrates, lipids, and proteins.

When the thyroid gland is overactive, the condition that develops is known as hyperthyroidism or Graves' disease. This is thought to be a disorder of the

THYRODIAGNOSTIC FLOWCHART

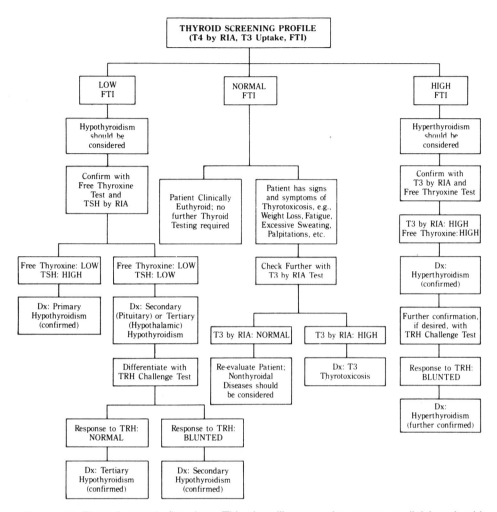

Figure 4.2. Thyrodiagnostic flowchart. This chart illustrates the process a clinician should undertake—from screening through diagnosis—when evaluating a patient's thyroid function.

autoimmune system and is much more prevalent among women than among men. Its occurrence may coincide with the following:

Disorders of carbohydrate metabolism (with abnormal blood glucose curves and glucose intolerance)
Increased protein metabolism
Calcium imbalance
Bone turnover caused by altered vitamin D metabolism
Disordered creatine metabolism
Depressed serum cholesterol and triglyceride levels
Accelerated vitamin requirements
Patient complaints of perspiration and heat intolerance
Slightly elevated basal body temperature
Acceleration of linear growth in children

As defined by Thilly et al. (6), the criteria for defining a goiter by stages are:

Grade 0   0a: Thyroid not palpable or, if palpable, not larger than normal.

0b: Thyroid distinctly palpable but usually not visible with the head in a normal or raised position, considered to be definitely larger than normal, at least as large as the distal phalanx of the subject's thumb.

Grade I Thyroid easily palpable and visible with the head in either a normal or raised position. The presence of a discrete nodule qualifies a patient for inclusion in this grade.

Grade II Thyroid easily visible with the head in a normal position.

Grade III Goiter visible at a distance.

Grade IV Monstrous goiters.

Conversely, when a patient exhibits deficient activity and reduced secretion of T3 and T4—or both—hypothyroidism may be present. It, too, usually is more prevalent in women than in men. (Often, this condition develops after treatment for hyperthyroidism.) Its occurrence may coincide with the following:

Flattened oral glucose tolerance curve (due to slowed absorption of glucose from the intestine)
Decreased conversion of carotene to vitamin A
Increased serum carotene levels
Rapid weight increase despite decreased appetite
Elevated blood cholesterol and triglyceride levels
Cold intolerance
Dry skin
Constipation
Lethargy
Decreased growth in children

Additionally, all or most of the following symptoms will be present in patients with severe hypothyroidism:

Physical/mental slowness
Decreased hearing
Thickened speech
Menorrhagia and sterility in menstruating women
Paresthesia of hands and feet
Cramping/aching of muscles

Comparison of Thyroid Function Tests

A number of methods are available to the clinician who wishes to analyze a patient's thyroid function in the laboratory. An examination of eight methods appears below. However, the practitioner also should remember the various cautions listed at the start of this section before initiating any of them and making a diagnosis based upon them.

1. T3 Uptake—The T3 Uptake test is not an assay for T3. Unfortunately, this test was named for the test reagent, the radiolabeled 3 reagent. T3 uptake tests are designed to assess the unsaturated binding capacity of certain serum proteins, primarily TBG. The classical definition of T3 uptake is the percentage of the total radioactivity added with the secondary binder.
2. T4 by RIA—In the past few years there has been a rapid escalation in the use of radioisotopic assays for thyroxine. The T4 assay is a quantitative measurement of total serum thyroxine.

3. Free Thyroxine Index (FTI)—The level of free T4 in serum is directly related to the two parameters that are easily and accurately measured by total T4 and the T3 uptake test. Because free T4 concentration is dependent upon the concentration of total T4 and the unsaturated TBG, close correlations have been demonstrated between the free T4 and the product of the total T4 and the T3 uptake. The product was termed Free Thyroxine Index and presently is the most widely accepted parameter of true thyroid status. Even in states in which TBG capacity is abnormal, thyroid status can be accurately assessed.
4. Thyroid-Binding Globulin (TBG)—This is the major transport for the thyroid hormones.
5. T3 by RIA—Triiodothyronine quantitation by RIA is based on the principle that endogenous T3 present in the serum sample and I-labeled T3 will compete equally for a constant but limited number of anti-T3 combining sites. Assessment of the labeled T3 allows quantitation of the unlabeled T3 present in the serum sample.
6. Free Triiodothyronine Index (FT3I)—Just as the total T4 levels are affected by varying concentrations of the thyroid hormone transport proteins, so too are T3 levels affected. In pregnancy and in patients taking oral contraceptives or estrogen, the increased TBG concentration elevates the total serum concentration. In cases of androgen therapy or hypoproteinemia, total T3 levels will be decreased. Multiplication of the T3 (RIA) result by the T3 Uptake test result provides an index that corresponds with the patient's thyrometabolic state.
7. Thyrotropin—Thyrotropin (the thyroid stimulating hormone, or TSH), a glycoprotein secreted by the anterior pituitary, regulates the secretion of thyroxine (T4) and triiodothyronine (T3) by the normal thyroid gland. TSH is in turn controlled by the level of free thyroxine hormone that is bound to thyrobinding proteins and by thyrotropin releasing hormone (TRH), which is released by the hypothalamus. Due to the negative feedback system between the thyroid and the pituitary, serum TSH reflects variations in the level of circulating free thyroid hormones.
8. Thyroid-Releasing Hormone—A thyrotropin-releasing hormone (or TRH) is produced by the hypothalamus and acts on the pituitary to stimulate the release of TSH. That portion involved in the control of TSH secretion is concentrated in the stalk-median eminence region of the hypothalamus. TRH is a tripeptide distributed throughout the brain. The pituitary response to TRH is extremely rapid. Intravenous administration of the TRH results in measurable increases in circulating TSH within 1 to 2 minutes. The hypothalamic secretion of TRH can be thought of as a "thermostat" regulating the upper and lower limits of T3 and T4, between which the pituitary-thyroid feedback mechanism will take place.

Malabsorption and Maldigestion Tests

There is considerable interlinking between the functions of digestion and absorption in the small intestine. The diagnosis of malabsorptive disease often is possible through the use of a few widely available tests. Patients with malabsorptive syndromes usually present themselves with either diarrhea or nutritional deficiencies, or both. The clinician should suspect malabsorption in any patient with diarrhea, even when the classic frothy, foul, floating, and greasy stools of steatorrhea are not present. In addition, the clinician must suspect malabsorption in anyone with unexplained nutritional deficiencies, even when there are no bowel symptoms. Deficiencies of iron and folate, vitamin B_{12} deficient anemias, bleeding disorders from vitamin K deficiencies, and osteomalacia also are typical.

Fat maldigestion is suggested by gross steatorrhea, and fecal fat excretion should be measured in such patients. Pancreatic dysfunction with subsequent fat maldigestion is tested by standard pancreatic secretion tests. Fat maldigestion also may be caused by bacterial overgrowth, which leads to deconjugation and dehydroxylation of bile acids. Carbohydrate maldigestion may be tested through the glucose tolerance test or by the measurement of the brush border enzyme activity in jejunal biopsy specimens. Protein maldigestion may be diagnosed by the peptide tolerance test. Jejunal biopsies also are important in excluding malabsorption states by demonstrating normal small intestinal mucosa.

Differentiating Between Maldigestion and Malabsorption

There are numerous methods that the clinician should employ to help determine the existence of maldigestion or malabsorption. For example, the practitioner may look first for the presence of any diseases or conditions that usually are associated with malabsorption (7). These include:

Disaccharidase deficiency
Tropical sprue
Nontropical sprue
Disorders of amino acid malabsorption
Abetalipoproteinemia
Vitamin B_{12} malabsorption
Monosaccharide malabsorption
Pancreatic insufficiency
Gastric acid hypersecretion
Gastric resection
Hepatobiliary disease
Interrupted enterohepatic circulation of bile salts
Endocrine and metabolic disorders
Mesenteric vascular insufficiency
Intestinal lymphangiectasia
Chronic congestive heart failure
Regional enteritis
Drug-induced enteritis
Infectious enteritis
Radiation enteritis
Ulcerative colitis
Amyloidosis
Scleroderma
Gastrointestinal allergy
Whipple's disease
Intestinal lymphoma

Various abnormalities that may be uncovered through a laboratory evaluation also are associated with malabsorption (8). These include:

Macrocytic, hyperchromic, hypochromic, or normochromic anemia (B_{12} and folic acid deficiency)
Microcytic, hypochromic anemia (iron and protein deficiency)
Hypocholesterolemia
Low prothrombin

Table 4.4
Differential Diagnosis of Malabsorption States

A number of tests are commonly used in the differential diagnosis of malabsorption states; by use of them the clinician can help determine whether the patient is suffering from malabsorption or maldigestion.

TESTS COMMONLY USED IN THE DIFFERENTIAL DIAGNOSIS OF MALABSORPTION STATES

	Malabsorption (e.g., sprue)	*Maldigestion* (e.g., pancreatic insufficiency)
1. *Stool exam*		
a. Fat—microscopic		
Neutral fat	N-↑	↑↑
Fatty acids	↑↑	↑
b. Fat—chemical—72 hour	↑	↑
c. 131ᵢ—Triolein excretion	↑	↑
d. 131ᵢ—Oleic acid excretion	↑	N
e. Undigested muscle fibers	N	↑
2. *Other parameters of fat and fat soluble vitamin absorption*		
a. Serum carotene, vitamin A	↓	↓
b. Serum prothrombin	↓	↓
c. Serum cholesterol	↓	↓
d. Serum calcium	↓	↓
3. *Carbohydrate absorption*		
a. Glucose tolerance	↓	N (occ. diabetic)
b. D-Xylose tolerance	↓	N (occ. ↓)
c. Lactose tolerance	may be ↓	N
4. *Schilling Test (B₁₂)*	Abn. (if ileal involvement)	N (occ. abn.)

Low serum calcium
Low serum phosphorous
Low serum potassium
Low serum albumin
Elevated alkaline phosphatase

The practitioner also may initiate a series of tests to help in the differentiation between the two conditions (see Table 4.4). Other tests that also may prove useful are listed below:

Maldigestion	*Malabsorption*
Jejunal biopsy	Glucose tolerance test
Fecal fat excretion	Serum alkaline phosphatase
D-xylose test	Straight x-ray of abdomen
Serum iron	Pancreatic function tests

Tests of Lipid Absorption

The qualitative analysis of fecal excretion of fat remains a useful but nonspecific test of overall digestive and absorptive functions of the small intestine. The standard method of measuring fat in the feces is one that measures fatty acids after hydrolysis of the extracted lipid. Patients with small intestinal malabsorption may or may not have steatorrhea. Normal fecal fat excretion does not exclude conditions such as celiac disease.

1. Tests of fat absorption using radioisotopes: The use of radioisotopes has long been a possibility in tests of lipid absorption. However, many problems have arisen with these tests.
2. Vitamin A and serum carotene measurements: A Vitamin A tolerance test may be helpful in determining the presence of malabsorption of lipids. The patient is fasted overnight and then given an oral dose of 180,000 I.U. of Vitamin A. Blood is taken every 2 hours for 8 hours, and serum vitamin A is measured.

   Carotene is the precursor to vitamin A, and its absorption also depends on normal fat transport. By measuring plasma carotene levels, the clinician will have another tool in the diagnosis of lipid malabsorption. Low plasma carotene levels may be present with normal vitamin A levels in some malabsorption states.
3. Plasma prothrombin time: The prothrombin time gives an indirect index of absorption of vitamin K. The prothrombin time may be prolonged when fat malabsorption is present.
4. Serum cholesterol: Serum cholesterol may be low in patients with small intestinal disease but is variable and a poor indication of the state of fat absorption.
5. Tests of vitamin D absorption: Vitamin D is a fat-soluble vitamin whose absorption may be affected in states of fat malabsorption. Plasma vitamin D levels can be measured by microbiological radioassay techniques, which yield measurements of the vitamin D metabolite 25-hydroxycholecalciferol.
6. Plasma vitamin E levels: Absorption of vitamin E parallels fat absorption. Vitamin E measurements can be used as an index of intestinal malabsorption although further testing is required.
7. Intestinal perfusion studies: The technique of intestinal perfusion recently has been applied to directly measure fat absorption in the small intestine. However, considerable technical problems remain due to the complexity of the perfusate and the use of markers.

Tests of Carbohydrate Absorption

1. D-xylose absorption test: This test is not in fact an adequate measure of carbohydrate absorption. However, the D-xylose absorption test has been regarded as an adequate means of screening for malabsorption and appears to reflect the effective surface area of the intestine rather than any specific absorption mechanism. A critical assessment of the D-xylose absorption test suggests that it has little purpose in routine practice and may give misleading results.
2. Oral glucose tolerance test (OGTT): The oral glucose tolerance test may be helpful in diagnosing malabsorption states. On occasion it can help pinpoint impaired absorption, which appears as a flat curve on the glucose tolerance test.

3. Lactose tolerance: This test may be used as a screening test for disaccharidase deficiency. However, it is less accurate than an assay of enzymes in small intestinal mucosa biopsies. If a significant lactose deficiency is present, the patient, upon ingestion of 50 gm lactose in 500 ml of water, will have symptoms including diarrhea, cramping, abdominal pain, and stomach distention. A flat curve on the lactose tolerance test suggests a monosaccharide malabsorption.

Protein

There are no satisfactory routine tests that accurately measure the absorption of dietary proteins or amino acids. Many patients with small intestinal disease and malabsorption have edema associated with hypoalbuminemia.

1. Plasma protein: Measurement of the serum proteins is useful. Hypoalbuminemia commonly occurs in small intestinal disease. Hypoglobulinemia together with hypoalbuminemia suggests a protein losing state in the intestine.
2. Fecal nitrogen: Measurement of fecal excretion of nitrogen provides indirect indication of protein absorption as it measures the residue of dietary and endogenous protein.

Tests for Protein-Losing Enteropathy

Tests for diagnosing excessive loss of protein into the lumen of the bowel are important in the clinical investigation of many patients. The techniques available make use of a number of radioisotopically labelled macromolecules. The ideal macromolecule is albumin as it is the principal protein lost in the lumen of the bowels.

Folic Acid

Malabsorption of folic acid is common in patients with diseases involving the upper intestine, such as celiac disease and Crohn's disease.

1. Serum folate and red cell folate levels: A deficiency of folic acid secondary to malabsorption can be rapidly identified by measuring serum folate.
2. Folate acid absorption test: Folic acid can be measured in blood samples after the oral administration of folic acid.

Vitamin B$_{12}$

A low serum vitamin B$_{12}$ is good evidence of a deficiency of the vitamin and may indicate a malabsorption problem.

For details about the Schilling test, see the section on nutritional anemias in Chapter 5.

Ascorbic Acid

Malabsorption of water-soluble ascorbic acid commonly occurs in generalized malabsorption states. Ascorbic acid deficiency can be determined by measuring the leukocyte ascorbic acid level. However, no specific absorption test of ascorbic acid is routinely administered.

Other B Vitamins

There is little known about malabsorption of thiamine, niacin, pyridoxine, and riboflavin in malabsorption syndromes. Although an increased excretion of tryptophan metabolites, xanthurenic acid, and kynurenic acid may give an indirect indication of a deficiency of pyridoxine, routine tests of absorption of the B vitamins are not in general use.

Iron

Tests for iron absorption are difficult to perform accurately, and the results are frequently difficult to interpret. The demonstration of a deficiency suggests the possibility of malabsorption of iron provided the dietary intake is adequate and blood loss can be excluded.

1. Serum iron and iron-binding capacity: A low serum iron with reduced iron binding capacity indicates the presence of iron deficiency.
2. Iron recovery in feces: After an overnight fast, the patient is given 59Fe as ferric chloride orally, and the stools are collected daily and counted for the presence and amount of radioactivity.

Tests of Calcium

These are not routinely used in clinical investigation. Apart from the basic biochemical tests aimed at identifying the presence of a calcium deficiency, specific tests of calcium absorption using radioisotopes or whole body counting are also available.

Tests of Magnesium, Zinc, Manganese

The trace minerals magnesium, zinc, and manganese have a considerable importance in normal body functions. Deficiencies of these elements are commonly associated with conditions giving rise to small intestinal malabsorption.

Deficiencies can be determined by measuring plasma levels of each of these minerals. Urinary excretion of 24-hour duration also should be measured.

References

1. Sauberlich HE, Dowdy RP, Skala JH. Laboratory tests for assessment of nutritional status. CRC Crit Rev Laboratory Sci 1973;4:3.
2. Brin M. Dilemma of marginal vitamin deficiency proc. IX Int Cong Nutr (Mexico City). 1972.
3. Statland BE, Winkel P. Effects of non-analytical factors on the intra-individual variation of analytes in the blood of healthy subjects: consideration of preparation of the subject and time of venipuncture. CRC Crit Rev Clin Lab Sci 1977(a);8:105.
4. Stout RW, Henry RW, Buchana KD. Triglyceride metabolism in acute starvation: the role of secretin and glucagon. Eur J Clin Invest 1976;6:170–185.
5. Freer DE, Statland BE. Effects of ethanol (0.75 g/kg body weight) on the activities of selected enzymes in sera of healthy young adults. Clin Chem 1977;23:830–834.
6. Thilly CH, Delange F, Stanbury JB. Epidemiologic surveys in endemic goiter and cretinism. In: Stanbury JB, Hetzel BS, eds. Endemic goiter and endemic cretinism. New York: John Wiley & Sons, 1980:157.
7. Krause MV, Mahan LK. Food nutrition and diet therapy: a textbook of nutritional care. 7th ed. Philadelphia: WB Saunders, 1984:451.
8. Ross JR, Moore VA. Axioms of malabsorption. Hosp Med 1975;11:98.

Suggested Readings

Alper C. Nutritional deficiencies: a laboratory mystery? The Condenser (Bio-science laboratories), 1973;4:4.

Baker H, Frank O, Hutner S. Vitamin analyses in medicine. In: Modern nutrition in health and disease. Philadelphia: Lea & Febiger, 1980.

Brin M. Dilemma of marginal vitamin deficiency proc. IX Int Cong Nutr (Mexico City). 1972.

Brin M. Biochemical assessment of nutritional status. In: Hawkins WW, ed. The assessment of nutritional status. Miles Laboratories Ltd, 1974.

Brin M. Red cell transketolase as an indicator of nutritional deficiency. Am J Clin Nutr 1980;33.

Butterworth CE, Blackburn GL. Hospital malnutrition and how to assess the nutritional status of a patient. Nutrition Today 1976;March–April.

Christakis G. Nutritional assessment in health programs. Am J Public Health 1973(Supplement, Nov);63.

Dix D, Cohen P, Kingsley S, Senkbeil J, Sexton K. Glycohemoglobin and glucose tolerance tests compared as indicators of borderline diabetes. Clin Chem 1979;25:877.

Engel RH, Pribor, H. C. Serum ferritin: a convenient measure of body iron stores. Laboratory Management 1978;October.

Freer DE, Statland BE. Effects of ethanol (0.75 g/kg body weight) on the activities of selected enzymes in sera of healthy young adults. Clin Chem 1977;23:830–834.

Gordon T. High-density lipoprotein as a protective factor against coronary artery disease: the Framingham study. Am J Med 1977;62:707–714.

Koenig RG. Correlation of glucose regulation and hemoglobin A1C and diabetes mellitus. N Engl J Med 1976;295:417–420.

Krause MV, Mahan LK. Food nutrition and diet therapy: a textbook of nutritional care. 7th ed. Philadelphia: WB Saunders, 1984.

Oates K. Laboratory measures of vitamin status. Laboratory Management 1980;May.

Ross JR, Moore VA. Axioms of malabsorption. Hosp Med 1975;11:98.

Sauberlich HE, Dowdy RP, Skala JH. Laboratory tests for assessment of nutritional status. CRC Crit Rev Lab Sci 1973;4:3.

Sauberlich HE. Laboratory indices of nutritional status. Nutrition and the M.D. 1979;5:5.

Shenkin A, Steele L. Clinical and laboratory assessment of nutritional status. Proc Nutr Society 1978;37.

Shils ME, Young VR, eds. Modern nutrition in health and disease. 7th ed. Philadelphia: Lea & Febiger, 1988.

Simko MD, Cowell C, Gilbride, JA. Nutrition assessment: a comprehensive guide for planning intervention. Rockville, Maryland: Aspen Publishers, 1984.

Stanbury JB, Hetzel BS, eds. Endemic goiter and endemic cretinism. New York: John Wiley & Sons, 1980.

Statland BE, Winkel P. Effects of non-analytical factors on the intra-individual variation of analytes in the blood of healthy subjects: consideration of preparation of the subject and time of venipuncture. CRC Crit Rev Clin Lab Sci 1977(a);8:105.

Stout RW, Henry RW, Buchana KD. Triglyceride metabolism in acute starvation: the role of secretin and glucagon. Eur J Clin Invest 1976;6:170–185.

Turkington RW, Weindling KK. Insulin secretion in the diagnosis of adult onset diabetes mellitus. JAMA 1978;240:833–836.

5

Drug-Nutrient Interactions

The interaction between food and drugs is a complicated process that is of great importance to any practitioner who plans to undertake a clinical assessment of nutritional status. Drugs that a patient may be ingesting, for example, may lead to a positive or negative impact on nutrient absorption, transport, metabolism, cellular uptake, and excretion. The changes they cause may be physiological or physiochemical. And adverse side effects may even result when dietary changes or related alterations of the patient's nutritional status have an impact on numerous drugs.

There are many ways that drugs and nutrients interact. Some of the most common of these include the following:

- Drugs can decrease the synthesis of certain vitamins and minerals.
- The use of particular drugs can decrease a patient's food intake by changing appetite and taste sensations and causing nausea.
- Some drugs cause malabsorption syndromes.
- Drugs may increase nutrient requirements.
- Drugs can block normal metabolism and promote excretion of nutrients.

It is recognized that these changes will be found more often in the elderly, in children, and in patients with chronic long-term disease. It is known that many of them develop slowly. And, quite often, the drugs responsible for a deficiency or the under-utilization of a particular nutrient will cause clinical symptoms that are easily recognized and noted. However, on other occasions, the symptoms will not be apparent and any effects that do develop must be uncovered through persistent questioning and careful analysis. It is imperative, therefore, that the clinician include a complete drug history in any nutritional assessment that is performed.

Moreover, there will be times when the practitioner determines that drugs alone are not responsible for a patient's poor nutritional status—unless, of course, the drugs were prescribed while the patient was on a suboptimal diet and the result is an exacerbation of various existing problems. These changes, instead, will likely develop from a variety of factors that may be having an impact on the patient simultaneously. These include a marginal nutritional status before drug prescription, the presence of catabolic disease, weight losses exceeding 10% of ideal body weight, and the traditionally poor dietary intake that regularly accompanies alcoholism and certain other conditions. All of this can be determined and duly noted during the history.

Additionally, the clinician should remember that any changes that do develop will come from a few well-known cause-and-effect processes. Food leads to various physiological alterations in the gastrointestinal tract, for instance, such as changes in gastric emptying; increased intestinal motility; increased splanchnic blood flow; increased bile, acid, and enzyme secretion; induction and inhibition of drug metabolism; and competition in active transport (1). All of these may be relevant when the potential interactions of food and drugs are being considered.

Potential effects of these interactions, quite obviously, can vary greatly due to a number of factors and therefore should be considered early and examined closely by the clinician. The following pages detail areas where these effects may be most severe, such as the impact of food and alcohol—separately and together—on drugs, the impact of drugs on food intake, the impact of drugs on nutrient absorption, and the impact of drugs on a patient's vitamin and mineral status. A thorough understanding of these effects will aid in the initiation of any nutritional assessment as well as the therapeutic process that will follow.

Effect of Food on Drugs

The absorption of drugs will either be increased or decreased by the physiological changes that take place during digestion. In some instances the absorption of a drug will be increased as a result of the nutrients in foods. In other cases the absorption of a drug will be decreased as a result of the nutrients in foods. This is particularly true in specific forms of dietary fiber that can absorb the drugs.

When the absorption of drugs is delayed, however, it does not necessarily mean that less of the drug is being absorbed. Instead, it means that the drug takes more time to reach peak blood levels. And it always should be remembered that drugs may not be as well absorbed when they are taken at the same time as food ingestion.

Drugs for Which Absorption is Delayed or Reduced by Food

Most drugs and most nutrients are absorbed in the small intestine, and so it is logical to assume that each may have an impact on the absorption of the other. This interaction is complex and dependent upon the dosage of the relevant drug, the type and amount of the food that is ingested, the timing of both actions, and the existence of any diseases.

Listed below are drugs for which absorption will be delayed by food intake:

Amoxicillin
Alclofenac
Cefaclor
Cephalexin
Cephradine
Cimetidine
Cinoxacin
Sulfadiazine
Sulfadiazine, sodium
Sulfafurazole (sulfisoxazole)
Sulfanilamide
Sulfadimethoxine
Sulfamethoxypyridazine
Sulfasymasine
Aspirin
Paracetamol (acetaminophen)

Indoprofen
Metronidazole
Digoxin
Diclofenac
Furosemide
Potassium ion
Glipizide
Phenytoin
Piroxicam
Quinidine
Theophylline

Those drugs for which absorption will be reduced by food intake are as follows:

Captopril
Cephalexin
Penicillin G
Penicillin V (K)
Penicillin V (Ca)
Penicillin V (acid)
Penicillamine
Phenethicillin
Phenylmercaptomethylpenicillin
Pivampicillin
Phenytoin
Ampicillin
Amoxicillin
Tetracycline
Demethylchlortetracycline
Demeclocycline (demethylchlortetracycline)
Methacycline
Oxytetracycline
Phenacetin
Phenazone (antipyrine)
Aspirin
Aspirin, calcium
Atenolol
Sotalol
Propantheline
Levodopa
Rifampin
Rifampicin
Doxycycline
Isoniazid
Hydrochlorothiazide
Phenobarbital
Ketoconazole
Lincomycin
Nafcillin
Theophylline

Drugs That Are Better Absorbed After Food Intake

Unlike those drugs listed above, there are many compounds that actually are absorbed more efficiently by the body after food has been ingested. Those drugs whose absorption is increased by food are:

Alafosfalin
Canrenone
Chlorothiazide
Hydrochlorothiazide
Dextropropoxyphene
Griseofulvin
Nitrofurantoin
Phenytoin
Diazepam
Dicoumarol
Diftalone
Lithium citrate
Alpha-tocopherol nicotinate
Riboflavin-5-phosphate
Riboflavin
Propranolol
Labetalol
Metoprolol
Hydralazine
Sulfamethoxydiazine
Spironolactone
Carbamazepine
Propoxyphene
Mebendazole
Methoxsalen
Pivampicillin

Changes in Diet That Affect the Rate of Drug Metabolism

Drug metabolism may be affected when nutritional deficiency is present, as well as when diet has been altered. Some of the factors to consider when attmepting to determine whether drug metabolism has been influenced include the following:

- Drugs may be metabolized faster on a high protein-low carbohydrate diet.
- Indolic compounds in cabbage, cauliflower, and brussel sprouts can increase the rate of drug metabolism.
- Polycyclic aromatic hydrocarbons (such as those produced by broiling foods over charcoal) are known to accelerate the metobolism of certain drugs like antipyrine, theophylline, phenacetin, and caffeine.

Adverse Drug Reactions Caused by Foods and Alcohol

Specific foods and/or alcoholic beverages can bring about adverse reactions to drugs. These reactions range from mild headaches to severe heart palpitations that can be life threatening (see Table 5.1).

Tyramine Reactions

When fermented foods like cheese are consumed by patients on monoamine oxidase inhibitor drugs—such as phenelzine (Nardil), isocarboxazid (Marplan), tranylcypromine (Parnate), procarbazine, and isoniazid—tyramine reactions may be noted in some patients. Because the absorption of tyramine may release catecholamines and result in elevated blood pressure in these patients, short

Table 5.1
Drug-Food and Drug-Alcohol Incompatibilities
The reactants and relevant effects for four classifications of reactions are listed.[a]

Classification	Reactants		Effect
	1	2	
1. Tyramine reactions	MAO/Inhibitors	High tyramine/dopamine foods	
	Antidepressants, e.g., phenelzine	Cheese	Flushing
		Red wines	Hypertension
	Procarbazine	Chicken Livers	Cerebrovascular accidents
	Isoniazid (INH, Isonicotinic acid hydrazide)	Broad beans Yeast extracts	
2. Disulfiram reactions	Aldehyde dehydrogenase inhibitors	Ethanol	Flushing, headache Nausea, vomiting Chest and abdominal pain
	Disulfiram (Antabuse)	Beer	
	Calcium carbamide	Wine	
	Metronidazole	Liquor	
	Sulfonylureas	Foods containing alcohol	
3. Hypoglycemic reactions	Insulin releasers	Ethanol	Weakness
	Oral hypoglycemic agents		Mental confusion
	Sugar (as in sweet mixes)		Irrational behavior Loss of consciousness
4. Flush reactions	Miscellaneous	Ethanol	Flush
	Chlorpropamide [+ diabetes]		Dyspnea
	Griseofulvin		Headache
	Tetrachloroethylene		

[a]From Roe DA. Interactions between drugs and nutrients. Med Clin N Am 1979;63(5):995–1011.

hypertensive attacks may develop. The reactions experienced by these patients are characterized by headaches, nausea, vomiting, palpitations, hypertension of short duration, and major cardiovascular attacks (occasionally).

Foods that are high in tyramine and may result in such a reaction are noted below, along with their tyramine content (2).

Foods/Beverages	Tyramine Content (Mg/g)
Cheese	
Cheddar	120–1500
Camembert	20–2000
Emmenthaler	225–1000
Stilton	466–2170
Processed	26–50
Brie	0–200
Gruyère	516
Gouda	20
Brick, natural	524
Mozzarella	410
Roquefort	27–520
Parmesan	4–290

Romano	238
Provolone	38
Cottage	5
Fish	
Salted, dried	0–470
Pickled herring	3000
Meat	
Meat extracts	95–304
Beef liver (stored)	274
Chicken liver (stored)	100
Vegetables	
Avocado	23
Fruit	
Banana	7
Alcoholic beverages	
Beer and ale	1.8–11.2
Wines	0–25
Chianti	25.4
Sherry	3.6

Hypoglycemic Reactions

When diabetic patients who are receiving oral hypoglycemic agents also ingest alcohol, a hypoglycemic reaction may result. Additionally, these reactions may be induced by foods that produce a rapid release of insulin into the bloodstream in combination with alcoholic beverages, as well as the consumption of alcohol with sweet mixes on an empty stomach.

Symptoms of a hypoglycemic reaction include weakness, mental confusion, irrational behavior, and loss of consciousness (if untreated).

Flush Reactions

In certain patients, flush reactions may be induced by a variety of drugs. These include:

Chlorpropamide (in certain diabetics)
Griseofulvin
Tetrachloroethylene
Central nervous system depressants in combination with alcohol
  Hypnotic sedatives
  Antihistamines
  Phenothiazines
  Narcotic analgesics

The symptoms that may accompany such a reaction are flushing (appears rapidly after ingestion of alcoholic beverages), dyspnea, and headaches.

Effect of Drugs on Food Intake and Absorption

Many drugs alter the appetite of the patient. Other drugs promote it. Sometimes these reactions can be used intentionally by the practioner, but in other cases they are an undesirable side effect and must be avoided. At all times, however, it is important to understand the impact that drugs may have on the patient's food intake and absorption. Drugs that both increase appetite (hyperphagic agents) and decrease appetite (hypophagic agents) are detailed below.

Hyperphagic Agents

1. Antihistamines—Cyproheptadine hydrochloride (Periactin)
2. Psychotropic drugs
   Chlorpromazine (Thorazine)
   Phenothiazines
   Benzodiazepines
   Chlordiazepoxide (Librium)
   Diazepam (Valium)
   Meprobamate
   Hydroxyzine hydrochloride (Atarax, Vistaril)
   Tricyclic antidepressants:
      Amitriptyline (Elavil)
      Combined tricyclic and monoamine oxidase inhibitor antidepressants
3. Hypoglycemic agents
   Insulin
   Sulfonylurea tolbutamide
   Chlorpropamide
4. Steroids
   Methandrostenolene (Dianabol)
   Nandrolone phenpropionate (Durabolin)
   Testosterone
   Glucocorticoids (most notable in patients with chronic adrenal insufficiency or anterior pituitary insufficiency)
   Antiinfective drugs, particularly tuberculostatic drugs in tuberculosis

Hypophagic Agents

1. Amphetamine and related stimulant drugs
   Fenfluramine (Pondimin)
   Dextroamphetamine (in hyperactive children)
   Methylphenidate (in hyperactive children)
2. Cancer chemotherapeutic drugs
   Methotrexate
   Purine derivatives
   Pyrimidine derivatives
3. Chelating agents
   D-Penicillamine and their side effects:
      Loss of taste (due to zinc deficiency)
      Diminished food intake
      Weight loss
4. Alcohol and its side affects:
   Anorexia
   Gastritis
   Lactose intolerance
   Pancreatitis
   Hepatitis
   Cirrhosis
   Alcoholic brain syndromes
   Ketoacidosis

Zinc deficiency
Protein deficiency
Riboflavin deficiency
Folic acid deficiency
Magnesium deficiency
Iron deficiency
Pantothenic acid deficiency
Copper deficiency
5. Cardiac glycosides
Digitalis, causing:
Anorexia
Nausea
Vomiting
Digitalis cachexia

Effect of Drugs on Nutrient Absorption

The use of many therapeutic drugs can lead to either primary or secondary malabsorption. Primary malabsorption comes as a direct result of drugs on the gastrointestinal tract. Secondary malabsorption comes when a drug interferes with the metabolism. In most situations dietary deficiencies of one nutrient can lead to malabsorption and deficiency of another nutrient.

Primary Intestinal Absorptive Defects Caused by Drugs

Listed below are nine drugs, their usage, the malabsorption or fecal nutrient loss they cause, and the mechanism involved (3).

1. Mineral Oil
Usage: Laxative
Malabsorption or fecal nutrient loss: carotene, vitamins A, D, K
Mechanism: Physical barrier, nutrients dissolve in mineral oil and are lost; micelle formation decreased
2. Phenolphthalein
Usage: Laxative
Malabsorption or fecal nutrient loss: vitamin D, Ca
Mechanism: intestinal hurry; K depletion; loss of structural integrity
3. Neomycin
Usage: Antibiotic to "sterilize" gut
Malabsorption or fecal nutrient loss: Fat, nitrogen, Na, K, Ca, Fe, lactose, sucrose, vitamin B_{12}
Mechanism: Structural defect; pancreatic lipase lowered; binding of bile acids (salts)
4. Cholestyramine
Usage: Hypocholesterolemic agent; bile acid sequestrant
Malabsorption or fecal nutrient loss: Fat, vitamins A, K, B_{12}, D, Fe
Mechanism: Binding of bile acids (salts) and nutrients, e.g., Fe
5. Potassium chloride
Usage: Potassium repletion
Malabsorption or Fecal Nutrient Loss: Vitamin B_{12}
Mechanism: Ileal pH lowered
6. Colchicine
Usage: Antiinflammatory agent in gout
Malabsorption or fecal nutrient loss: Fat, carotene, Na, K, vitamin B_{12}, lactose

Mechanism: Mitotic arrest; structural defect; enzyme damage
7. Biguanides—Metformin; Phenformin
    Usage: Hypoglycemic agents (in diabetes)
    Malabsorption or fecal nutrient loss: vitamin B_{12}
    Mechanism: Competitive inhibition of B_{12} absorption
8. Paraamino—salicylic acid
    Usage: Antituberculosis agent
    Malabsorption or fecal nutrient loss: Fat, folacin, vitamin B_{12}
    Mechanism: Mucosal block in B_{12} uptake
9. Salicylazo-sulfapyridine (Azulfidine)
    Usage: Antiinflammatory agent in ulcerative colitis, and regional enteritis
    Malabsorption or fecal nutrient loss: Folacin
    Mechanism: Mucosal block in folate uptake

Drugs Causing Secondary Malabsorption

There also are several drugs that can result in secondary malabsorption. Seven of them, their usage, the resultant malabsorption, and the mechanism involved, are listed below (4).

1. Prednisone (other glucocorticoids)
    Usage: Used in allergic and collagen
    Malabsorption: Calcium
    Mechanism: Calcium transport decreased
2. Phenobarbital
    Usage: Anticonvulsant
    Malabsorption: Calcium
    Mechanism: Accelerated metabolism of vitamin D
3. Diphenylhydantoin
    Usage: Anticonvulsant
    Malabsorption: Calcium
    Mechanism: Accelerated metabolism of vitamin D
4. Primodone
    Usage: Anticonvulsant
    Malabsorption: Calcium
    Mechanism: Accelerated metabolism of vitamin D
5. Glutethimide
    Usage: Sedative
    Malabsorption: Calcium
    Mechanism: Impaired Ca transport
6. Diphosphonates
    Usage: Paget's disease
    Malabsorption: Calcium
    Mechanism: 1, 25-(OH)2-D3 formation
7. Methotrexate
    Usage: Leukemia
    Malabsorption: Calcium
    Mechanism: Acute folacin deficiency

Effect of Drugs on Vitamin and Mineral Status

Vitamin and mineral depletion or deficiency can be induced by a number of therapeutic drugs, as well as by various drug-nutrient interactions. These may be utilized intentionally by the practioner, or they may occur as an unwanted side effect of a prescribed drug therapy.

Drugs that interfere with the metabolism and physiological effect of vitamins are called vitamin antagonists. These specific drugs, along with their nutritional interactions and the clinical significance of same, are listed below. Additionally, certain therapeutic drugs can have an impact on mineral status by resulting in overload or depletion. These drugs, their interactions and significance also are detailed below.

Analgesics

1. Nonnarcotic salicylates, aspirin

Nutritional Interaction	*Clinical Significance*
Decreased platelet level of vitamin C.	Can cause hypoprothrombinemia and lengthen bleeding time.
Iron deficiency.	
Folate deficiency.	Increased numbers of deformed babies born to mothers on salicylates.
Malabsorption of glucose and xylose.	High doses cause gastrointestinal (GI) disturbances. Can produce GI bleeding, especially with alcohol.

Anorexic Agents

1. Amphetamines: Benzadrine, Dexedrine, Desoxyn, Dexamil

Nutritional Interaction	*Clinical Significance*
Decreases appetite.	Suppresses growth in young children.
Gastric irritant (Dexamil).	

Antacids

1. All antacids

Nutritional Interaction	*Clinical Significance*
Destruction of thiamine.	Occurs mainly with chronic use (i.e., hourly).
Decrease in absorption of iron.	
Increase in amount of sodium in the body.	Can cause fluid retention.

Aluminum Antacids

1. Maalox, Gelusil, Amphojel, Mylanta

Nutritional Interaction	*Clinical Significance*
Decreases absorption of phosphate.	May cause hypophosphatemia, hypercalciuria, hypomagnesemia, osteomalacia, renal stones.
Decreases the absorption of vitamin A.	May induce constipation.

2. Calcium-containing antacids

Nutritional Interaction	*Clinical Significance*
Decreased absorption of phosphate.	Hypophosphatemia.

3. Sodium bicarbonate

Nutritional Interaction	*Clinical Significance*
Decreased absorption of magnesium. Increased sodium in the body. Possibly decreased absorption of iron.	Can cause steatorrhea or magnesium. May cause edema. Significant only in large doses.

Antibiotics

1. Amphotericin

Nutritional Interaction	*Clinical Significance*
Increases the excretion of magnesium, phosphate, potassium.	Can cause hypokalemia, hypomagnesemia, hypophosphatemia.

2. Chloramphenicol

Nutritional Interaction	*Clinical Significance*
Increases the iron in the serum. Decreases folate, vitamin B_{12} and hemotopoietic response. Decreases absorption of glucose and amino acids.	Anemia often seen.

3. Cycloserine

Nutritional Interaction	*Clinical Significance*
Decreases folate in serum. Deficiency of pyridoxine.	May see neurological symptoms of pyridoxine deficiency.

4. Ethambutol

Nutritional Interaction	*Clinical Significance*
Zinc and/or copper metabolism is altered.	

5. Gentamicin, capreomycin, tobramycin, viomycin

Nutritional Interaction	*Clinical Significance*
Increases the excretion of calcium, magnesium, and possibly phosphate.	Severe electrolyte disturbances.

6. Isoniazid

Nutritional Interaction	*Clinical Significance*
Pyridoxine deficiency.	Neuritis that may be incapacitation. The malnourished and alcoholics are more susceptible to deficiencies.

7. Kanamycin, Neomycin, Paromomycin

Nutritional Interaction	*Clinical Significance*
Decreases the absorption of vitamins A, D, K, B_{12}. Decreases the absorption of sodium, potassium, iron, calcium. Decreases absorption of fat, cholesterol, sugar, protein.	Can cause significant malabsorption with chronic therapy.

CUT HERE

8. Paraaminosalicylic acid (PAS)

Nutritional Interaction	*Clinical Significance*
Decreases absorption of B_{12}, folate, cholesterol, xylose.	Malabsorption
	Megaloblastic anemia.
Decrease in vitamin K coagulation factors.	Only with those patients taking anticoagulants.
Increased excretion of potassium.	Hypokalemia.
Can cause deficiency of pyridoxine.	

9. Penicillin

Nutritional Interaction	*Clinical Significance*
Delayed absorption when taken with food.	
May cause malabsorption of vitamin B_{12}, calcium, magnesium, glucose, carotene and cholesterol.	
May decrease vitamin K synthesis.	
May decrease folate utilization and inactivates pyridoxine.	

10. Tetracycline

Nutritional Interaction	*Clinical Significance*
Decreases absorption of calcium, iron, magnesium, copper, cobalt, manganese, zinc.	Most common in long-term oral therapy in combination with low dietary intake of vitamin K. Often seen in patients on anticoagulants.
Decreases the vitamin K-dependent coagulation factors.	
Decreases leukocyte ascorbic acid level.	
Can cause deficiency of riboflavin, pyridoxine, vitamin B_{12}.	
Decreases level of pantothenic acid in serum.	
Can cause weight loss.	

Anticoagulants

1. Sodium Warfarin; Coumadin

Nutritional Interaction	*Clinical Significance*
Decreases vitamin K-dependent factors.	The likelihood of a deficiency increases when there is a deficiency of potassium, ascorbic acid, and dietary fat.
Prothrombin time decreases if the patient also is taking griseofulvin.	

Anticonvulsants

1. Phenobarbital, diphenylhydantoin

Nutritional Interaction	*Clinical Significance*
Accelerated vitamin D metabolism.	Rickets in children, osteomalacia in adults.

Decreased calcium absorption.
Accelerated vitamin K metabolism.
Low serum levels of folate, especially
    after 5 years or more of therapy.   Can cause mental disturbances and
Hypomagnesemia in epileptics who   neuropathy.
    take anticonvulsants.   Gastric irritant.
Possible vitamin B_{12} deficiency if
    intake has been low.   Effect altered with alcohol.

Antidiabetic Agents

1. Insulin

Nutritional Interaction	*Clinical Significance*
	May be teratogenic, no definite proof if defects are due to nutritional causes.

2. Sulfonylureas, tolbutamide, chlorpropamide, tolazamide, acetohexamide

Nutritional Interaction	*Clinical Significance*
Malabsorption of xylose, glucose.	Gastric irritant. Antabuse-like reaction if taken in combination with alcohol.

3. Biguanides; Phenformin

Nutritional Interaction	*Clinical Significance*
Malabsorption of vitamin B_{12}, calcium, amino acids, glucose, xylose, fat, water, electrolytes.	Gastric irritant. Taste acuity is altered.

Antihyperlipemics

1. Colestipol; Colestid

Nutritional Interaction	*Clinical Significance*
Malabsorption of vitamins A, D, E, K.	

2. Cholestyramine; Questran

Nutritional Interaction	*Clinical Significance*
Decreased absorption of vitamins A, B_{12}. Decreased absorption of iron, electrolytes, xylose. Vitamin K deficiency with prolonged use in high doses. Decreases vitamin K-dependent factors.	Constipation can occur.

3. Clofibrate; Atromid-S

Nutritional Interaction	*Clinical Significance*
May decrease the absorption of vitamin B_{12}, iron, carotene, glucose, electrolytes, medium chain triglycerides, and xylose.	Weight gain, nausea, diarrhea, altered taste sensations.

Antiinflammatory Agents

1. Colchicine

Nutritional Interaction   *Clinical Significance*
Decreases absorption of vitamins A,
D, B$_{12}$, fat, xylose, lactose.

2. Salicylates

Nutritional Interaction   *Clinical Significance*
Decreases vitamin K-dependent coagu-   Seen only when used in high doses
lation factors.   over a long period of time. Un-
                                        common.

Antineoplastics

1. Acitinomycin D, Mithramycin

Nutritional Interaction   *Clinical Significance*
Decreases absorption of calcium.   Hypocalcemia (a desired therapeutic
                                    effect of mithramycin).

2. Cyclophosphamide

Nutritional Interaction   *Clinical Significance*
Decreases absorption of fat   Can cause severe steatorrhea
                                    (although uncommon).
Decreases absorption of thiamine.

3. Methotrexate

Nutritional Interaction   *Clinical Significance*
Causes deficiency of folate.   Toxicity is enhanced if there is an exist-
                                    ing deficiency of folate and Vitamin
                                    B$_{12}$.

Decreased absorption of vitamin B$_{12}$,
carotene, fat, cholesterol, lactose,
xylose.

Cardiovascular Preparations

1. Digitalis: Cardiac glycosides, Acylanid, Digitaline, Lanoxin

Nutritional Interaction   *Clinical Significance*
Increases rate of excretion of   Either hypercalcemia or hypokalemia
  calcium, magnesium.   can induce toxicity.
Decrease in absorption of glucose
  and xylose.
Magnesium deficiency increases
  sensitivity to drugs.

2. Nitroglycerin

Nutritional Interaction   *Clinical Significance*
Hypotension can be induced with
  consumption of alcohol.

Corticosteroids

1. Cortisone, prednisone

Nutritional Interaction	*Clinical Significance*
Increases metabolism of vitamin D.	Can cause muscle weakness.
Increased excretion of vitamin C, zinc, potassium, magnesium.	Can cause delayed wound healing (from inadequate zinc) and muscle weakness from inadequate potassium.
Increased need of vitamin B_6.	May cause abnormalities of glucose tolerance.

Diuretics

1. Chlorothiazide

Nutritional Interaction	*Clinical Significance*
Increases the excretion of potassium.	Can cause muscle weakness.
Increases the excretion of magnesium leading to depletion.	Can induce hypoglycemia or aggravate diabetes.
Increased excretion of zinc, iodine.	May induce gout.

Hypotensives

1. Hydralazine

Nutritional Interaction	*Clinical Significance*
Can cause vitamin B_6 depletion.	Can bring on symptoms of polyneuritis.

Laxatives

1. Mineral Oil

Nutritional Interaction	*Clinical Significance*
Decreases absorption of vitamins A, D, E, K and electrolytes.	Regular ingestion during pregnancy can cause hypothrombinemia.
Decreased absorption of calcium.	

Oral Contraceptive Agents

Nutritional Interaction	*Clinical Significance*
Decreases folate in the serum	Megaloblastic anemia may be seen.
Pyridoxine deficiency.	
Decreased vitamin B_{12}.	Depression, weight gain.
May be increased need for riboflavin.	
Increased plasma vitamin A, increased serum vitamin E, increased copper absorption.	
Triglycerides, hemoglobin, and hematocrit are increased.	

Parkinsonian Drugs

1. Levodopa, Dopar

Nutritional Interaction	*Clinical Significance*
Drug effect reduced by high protein intake.	GI disturbances.

2. Larodopa

Nutritional Interaction
Pyridoxine interferes with drug
action.
Decreased absorption of glucose,
xylose.

Clinical Significance
Possible weight loss and taste
changes.

3. Procyclidine; Kemadrin

Nutritional Interaction

Clinical Significance
Gastric irritant.

4. Trihexyphenidyl; Artane

Nutritional Interaction

Clinical Significance
Gastric irritant. Causes dryness in
mouth.

Sedatives

1. Barbiturates, Amytal, Nembutal, Seconal

Nutritional Interaction
Increases the requirement for
vitamin C
Can cause deficiency of vitamin D
and folate.
Effect altered with alcohol.

Clinical Significance

References

1. Neuvonen PJ, Kivisto KT. The clinical significance of food-drug interactions: a review. Med J Australia 1989;150:36.
2. Roe DA. Interactions between drugs and nutrients. Med Clin North Am 1979;63(5):995–1011.
3. Roe DA. Interactions between drugs and nutrients. Med Clin North Am 1979;63(5):995–1011.
4. Roe DA. Interactions between drugs and nutrients. Med Clin North Am 1979;63(5):995–1011.

Suggested Readings

Adams PW, Rose DP. Effect of pyridoxine hydrochloride (vitamin B_6) upon depression associated with oral contraception. Lancet 1973;1:897–904.
Avioli LV, Birge SJ. Effects of prednisone on vitamin D metabolism in man. J Clin Endocrinol Metab 1968;28:1341–1346.
Baker LR. Iatrogenic osteomalacia and myopathy due to phosphate depletion. Br Med J 1974;3:150–152.
Bowden AN. Anticonvulsants and calcium metabolism. Develop Med Child Neurol 1974;16:214–217.
Cambell TC, Hayes JR. Role of nutrition in the drug metabolizing enzyme system. Pharmacol Rev 1974;26:171–197.
Coffey G, Wilson CW. Ascorbic acid deficiency and aspirin induced haematemesis. Br Med J 1975;1:208.
D'arcy PF, Griffin JP. Iatrogenic diseases. London: Oxford University Press, 1972.
Dent CE, Richens A. Osteomalacia with long term anticonvulsant therapy in epilepsy. Br Med J 1970;4:69–72.

Duarte GC, Winnacker JL. Thiazide-induced hypercalcemia. New Engl J Med 1971; 284:828–830.

Evered DF. L-dopa as a vitamin B_6 antagonist. Lancet 1971;1:914. Faloon WW. Effect of neomycin and kanamycin upon intestinal absorption. Ann NY Acad Sco 1966;132:879–887.

Finkelstein W, Isselbacher KJ. Drug therapy: cimetidine. New Engl J Med 1978;299:992–996.

Fitzgerald MG. Alcohol sensitivity in diabetics receiving chlorpropamide. Diabetes 1962;2:40.

Haghshenass M, Rao DB. Serum folate levels during anticonvulsant therapy with diphenylhydantoin. J Am Geriat Soc 1973;21:275–277.

Hahn TJ, Birge SJ. Phenobarbital-induced alterations in vitamin D metabolism. J Clin Invest 1972A;51:741–748.

Hodge JV, Nye ER. Monoamine oxidase inhibitors, broad beans and hypertension. Lancet 1964;1:1108.

Horwitz D, Lowenberg W. Monoamine oxidase inhibitors, tyramine and cheese. J Am Med Assoc 1964;188:1108–1110.

Jones CC. Megaloblastic anemia associated with long-term tetracycline therapy. Ann Intern Med 1973;78:910–912.

Kimberg DV. Effects of vitamin D and steroid hormones on the active transport of calcium by the intestine. New Engl J Med 1969;28:1396–1405.

Krause MV, Mahan LK. Food, nutrition and diet therapy: a textbook of nutritional care. 7th ed. Philadelphia: WB Saunders Company, 1984.

Leonards JR, Levy G. Gastrointestinal blood loss during prolonged aspirin administration. New Engl J Med 1973;289:1020–1022.

Lim P, Jacob E. Magnesium deficiency in patients on long-term diuretic therapy for heart failuire. Br Med J 1972;3:620–22.

Livingston S, Berman W. Anticonvulsant drugs and vitamin metabolism. J Am Med Assoc 1973;244:1634–1635.

Longenecker JB, Basu SG. Effect of cholestyramine on absorption of amino acids and vitamin A in man. (Abstract) Fed Proc 1965;24:375.

Manner RJ, Brechbill DO. Prevelance of hypokalemia in diuretic therapy. Clin Med 1972;79:19–22.

McWhirter WR. Ascorbic acid and long-term steroids. Lancet 1974;2:776.

Nardone DA, McDonald WJ. Mechanisms of hypokalemia: clinical correlations. Medicine 1978;57:435–446.

Necheles TF, Snyder LM. Malabsorption of folate polyglutamate associated with oral contraceptive therapy. New Engl J Med 1970;282:858–859.

Neubauer C. Mental deterioration in epilepsy due to folate deficiency. Br Med J 1970;2:759–761.

Neuvonen PJ, Gothoni G. Interference of iron with the absorption of tetracyclines in man. Br Med J 1970;4:532–534.

Neuvonen PJ, Matilla M. Interference of iron and milk with absorption of tetracycline. Scand J Clin Lab Invest (Suppl) 1971;27:76.

Neuvonen PJ, Kivisto KT. The clinical significance of food-drug interactions: a review. Med Australia 1989;150:36.

Newman LJ, Lopez R. Riboflavin deficiency in women taking oral contraceptive agents. Am J Clin Nutr 1978;31:247–249.

O'Keefe SJ, Marx V. Lunch-time gin and tonic: A cause of reactive hypoglycemia. Lancet 1977;1:1286–87.

Paykel PS. Amitriptyline, weight gain and carbohydrate craving: a side effect. Br J Psychiatry 1973;123:501–503.

Prasad AS. Effect of oral contraceptive agents on nutrients: I. Minerals. Am J Clin Nutr 1975B;28:377–384.

Prasad AS. Effect of oral contraceptive agents on nutrients: II. Vitamins. Am J Clin Nutr 1975B;28:385–391.

Pyke DA, Leslie RD. Chlorpropamide-alcohol flushing: a definition of its relation to non-insulin-dependent diabetes. B Med J 1978;2:1521–1522.

Reynolds EH. Mental effects of anticonvulsants and folic acid metabolism. Brain 1968;91:197–214.

Roe DA. Minireview: effects of drugs on nutrition. Life Sci I 1974;15:1219–1234.

Roe DA. Drug-induced nutritional deficiencies. Westport, Connecticut: The AVI Publishing Co., 1978.

Roe DA. Interactions between drugs and nutrients. Med Clin North Am 1979;63(5):995–1011.

Roe DA. Nurtient and drug interactions. Nutr Rev 1984;4:141–154.

Sanpitak N, Chayutimonkul L. Oral contraceptives and riboflavin nutrition. Lancet 1974;1:836–837.

Seixas FA. Alcohol and its drug interactions. Ann Intern Med 1975;83:86–92.

Shields HM. Rapid fall of serum phosphorus secondary to antacid therapy. Gastroenterology 1978;75:1137–1141.

Shils ME, Young VR, eds. Modern nutrition in health and disease. 7th ed. Philadelphia: Lea & Febiger, 1988.

Smith J, Goldsmith G. Effects of oral contraceptive steriods on vitamin and lipid levels in serum. Am J Clin Nutr 1975;28:371.

Stamp TC. Effects on long-term anticonvulsant therapy on calcium and vitamin D metabolism. Proc R Soc Med 1974;67:64–68.

Standall BR, Kao-Chen SM. Early changes in pyridoxine status of patients receiving isoniazid therapy. Am J Clin Nutr 1974;27:479–484.

Tolman KG, Jubiz W. Rickets associated with anticonvulsant medications (Abstract) Clin Res 1972;20:414.

Welling P. Nutrient effects on drug metabolism and action in the elderly. Drug-Nutr Interact 1985;4(1/2):187.

Zakim D, Herman RH. Clofibrate induced changes in the activity of human intestinal enzymes. Gastroenterology 1969;56:496–499.

6

Special Topics

A variety of special nutrition-related situations may present themselves to the practitioner who is in the process of assessing a patient's nutritional status. These special situations—although certainly unique to each individual involved—nonetheless can be divided into several general categories that then permit the clinician to more efficiently identify their related nutritional side effects and to more effectively plan an appropriate treatment program. When any of these situations is uncovered, therefore, it demands special attention.

The conditions (or special topics) to be discussed fully in the following pages include childhood and adolescence, pregnancy, obesity and exercise, anorexia nervosa, athletic performance, the musculoskeletal system, food allergies, anemias, the immune system, cardiovascular disease, geriatrics and degenerative disease, and the hospitalized patient. Each of these will have an impact on the nutritional status of the patient who exhibits it, and any that exist should be considered fully by the clinician when signs of it are uncovered during early stages of the assessment procedure.

The rapid growth rate of children and various nutritional deficiencies of the elderly, for two common and obvious examples, must be taken into account by anyone dealing with the mental and physical development of members of these two populations. However, perhaps less obviously, patients who show signs of any of the other conditions that are mentioned above also will have their own particular nutrition requirements that must be carefully considered and completely addressed when appropriate.

To help determine the unique nutritional peculiarities that are associated with each of these special topics, the clinician should focus on a number of specific questions when administering a case history to patients who seem to fit into the relevant categories. Likewise, various well-defined signs also will become apparent during the physical examination and the dietary history of affected individuals. And still other symptoms may be uncovered through anthropometric measuring or laboratory testing.

A thorough understanding of the impact that each of these special conditions may have on nutritional status—as well as the manner in which each can show up during a comprehensive nutritional assessment—will enable the practitioner to render a more accurate evaluation of the patient's individual situation. Ultimately, this knowledge also will aid in the initiation of the most beneficial therapeutic course of action possible.

Childhood and Adolescence

Any practitioner who assesses the nutritional status of infants, children, and adolescents will face a challenging and exciting task. The first 2 years of life are marked by rapid physical growth and social development, both of which bring with them a variety of changes in dietary practices and nutrient intake. From the second birthday until the onset of puberty, these changes continue in a less dramatic—but no less significant—fashion. And then comes adolescence, when physical and psychological changes once again become intense.

A nutritional assessment of youngsters, therefore, entails paying particular attention to their increasing physical stature and the numerous alterations in organ size and body function that accompany this growth. The clinician must remember that all of these normally occurring changes will contribute to an increased metabolic need for nutrients, as well as various parameters that must be carefully examined in order to eliminate any nutritional deficiencies that might develop.

Even among this overall population, moreover, special conditions also may be present that demand special attention. For infants, these can include low birth weight, the presence of specific diseases, the development of feeding skills, and the course of developmental growth. For children, they include physical growth patterns, developmental progress, dietary habits, the presence of specific diseases, and dental development. For adolescents, the focus is on physical and psychological development, sexual maturity, dietary habits, eating disorders, physical fitness and athletic practices, and behavioral problems.

Special Considerations: Case History

Child's weight at birth
Breast or bottle fed
Present weight/height
Any recent weight loss/gain
Does/did the child have any of the following:
  Birth trauma
  Colic
  Constipation
  Diarrhea
  Vomiting
  Anemia
  Anorexia
  Obesity
  Marasmus
  Kwashiorkor
  Lactos intolerance
  Gluten intolerance
  Allergies
  Asthma
  Dyslexia
  Food poisoning
Problems with motor coordination
Problems with learning, concentration
Impaired sexual development
What are the child's eating habits?
  Is the child fed on a rigid schedule?
  Does the child have digestive problems?

Gas
Bloating
Indigestion
Inability to eat
Excessive appetite
Does the child get along with parents?
Are there major problems with discipline?
Is "food" used as a reward? A punishment?
Is the child able to relate to the parents with warmth and affection?
Are the parents able to relate to the child with warmth and affection?
Does the child use food as a weapon against the parents?
Is there parental support for nutritional modifications?
Are there any metabolic disorders?
Inborn errors of metabolism
Renal disease
Liver disease
Heart disease
Hypercholesterolemia
Failure to thrive
Constant colds and infections
Kidney disease
Cystic fibrosis
Endocrine disorders

Special Considerations: Dietary History

Vitamin A deficiency:
Xerophthalmia
Keratomalacia
Bitot's spots
Night blindness
Vitamin B_1:
Infantile beriberi
Vitamin B_2:
Deficiency may occur during rapid growth in childhood
Angular stomatitis
Vitamin B_3:
Dermatitis
Neurological abnormalities
Vitamin C:
Scurvy
In infants:
Poor appetite
Irritability
Minimal growth
Tenderness of legs
Pseudoparalysis of lower extremities
Bleeding of skin and gums
Hemorrhages all over the body
Petechiae
Costochondral beading
Changes in cartilage shaft junction at sternal ends of ribs, distal end of the femur, and proximal end of the humerus

Vitamin D:
> In infants:
>> Tetany
>> Convulsions (rarely seen before 3 to 4 months of age)
>> Rickets
>> Progressive bony deformities from mechanical weakness of bone
>> Craniotabes
>> Enlargement of costochondral junctions of ribs produce "rachitic rosary"
>> Harrison's groove
>> Growing ends of long bones and ankles are widened at wrists and ankles
>> Deformities of pelvis
>> Scoliosis of spine
>> Teeth delayed in the eruption and enamel is defective

Special Considerations: Physical Examination

The clinician examining the child must be especially alert for various signs indicative of nutritional deficiencies. Each of these clinical symptoms is fully explained in Chapter 1.

Hair
> Flag sign

Face
> Moon face

Eyes
> Conjunctival xerosis
> Corneal xerosis
> Bitot's spots
> Keratomalacia

Lips
> Angular stomatitis
> Cheilosis

Tongue
> Magenta colored
> Glossitis

Teeth
> Caries

Gums
> Spongy

Musculoskeletal
> Muscle wasting
> Craniotabes
> Frontal and parietal bossing

Pregnancy

There are a number of factors that, alone and together, will have an impact on the course and the outcome of a pregnancy. These include the mother's age and physical condition, any traits she has inherited, any illnesses or infections she may contract, any adverse physical habits she may have (like smoking or substance abuse), and any exposure to toxic materials. Additionally—and of primary concern to the practitioner who is undertaking an assessment of nutritional status—the mother's dietary intake and nutrition habits certainly will have a profound effect.

During pregnancy, a mother to be will undergo tremendous physiological and biochemical changes in order for fetal growth and development to take place. These processes alter the woman's metabolic needs and make it more difficult for her to maintain her own homeostasis while also providing for the growing fetus. The nutritional status of the mother throughout pregnancy, therefore, is of crucial importance to the health of both the mother and the child. It also is a variable that a woman and the practitioner are capable of monitoring and controlling.

Areas that should be watched closely when assessing the nutritional status of a pregnant woman are her physiological changes (including prepregnancy weight and maternal weight gain), dietary habits, nutrition knowledge, caffeine and alcohol use, the presence of diseases or complications, and the intake of protein, vitamins, and minerals.

Special Considerations: Case History

Age of mother
Prepregnancy weight
Weight gain
Pattern of weight accumulation
Concern with body image
Change in eating habits
Strict vegetarianism (no milk, eggs, poultry, meat, fish)
Cravings
Nausea
Vomiting
Tiredness
Nervousness
Stress
Fatigue
Boredom
Decreased physical activity
Level of education
Level of income
Lack of knowledge about pregnancy-related needs
Previous obstetric history
   Spontaneous abortion
   Delivery of low birth weight infant
   Frequent pregnancies
Food allergies
Personal habits
   Alcohol
   Tobacco
Medications
   Prescription
   Nonprescription

Special Considerations: Dietary History

Iron: Dietary iron generally inadequate for pregnancy
   Increased need due to:
      Increased maternal circulating blood volume
      Increased hemoglobin
      Fetal liver iron storage

High iron cost of pregnancy

Folate
  Increased need due to:
    Increased metabolic demand of pregnancy
    Increased heme production
    Production of cell nucleus material
  Deficiencies result in:
    Megaloblastic anemia
    Spontaneous abortions
    Possible fetal malformations
    Preeclampsia

Calcium
  Increased need due to:
    Fetal skeletal formation
    Fetal tooth bud metabolism
    Increased maternal calcium metabolism
  Deficiencies result in:
    Maternal deficiency of calcium and vitamin D with complications of early
      neonatal hypocalcemia
    Possible leg cramping

Vitamin B$_6$ (pyridoxine)
  Increased need due to:
    Increased fetal growth requirement
    Increased protein in the diet
  Deficiency may result in:
    Preeclampsia
    Altered glucose metabolism

Vitamin B$_{12}$
  Increased need due to:
    Formation of red blood cells
    Coenzyme in protein metabolism especially nucleic acid
  Deficiency results in:
    Megaloblastic anemia
    Damage to nervous system

Sodium
  Until recently women were advised to decrease sodium intake. However,
    recent studies have indicated that inadequate sodium intake leads to hypo-
    valemia and to compensatory vasospasm. At the present time there is no
    convincing rationale for sodium restriction in normal pregnancy.

Niacin and riboflavin
  Increased need due to:
    Coenzyme in protein and energy metabolism
    Increased calorie intake
  Deficiency can result in:
    Nervousness

Vitamin A
  Increased need due to:
    Tissue growth
    Tooth bud formation in fetus
  Overabundance can result in congenital renal anomalies

Protein
  Increased need due to:
    Rapid fetal tissue growth
    Placenta growth and development

Maternal tissue growth in uterus, breasts
Increased maternal storage reserves for labor, delivery, lactation
Deficiency results in:
Restriction in critical period of development of the fetus results in the adult brain having fewer cells than if maternal diet were not restricted

Special Considerations: Physical Examination

Diabetes
Obesity
Heart disease
Edema (except in lower extremities)
Changes in hair color or texture
Hair loss
Pallor
Glossitis
Ataxia
Koilonychia
Seborrheic dermatitis
Alopecia

Special Considerations: Laboratory Examination

There are several types of anemia that can occur during pregnancy. These include:

Iron deficiency
Folic acid deficiency
Megaloblastic anemia
Anemia from blood loss
Anemia from infection
Acquired hemolytic anemia
Aplastic or hypoplastic anemia
Hereditary anemias: thalassemia, sickle cell anemia

There are several types of toxemias that can occur during pregnancy. These include:

Hypertensive
Proteinuria
Edema

Obesity and Exercise

Obesity and exercise are two topics of related concern during an assessment of nutritional status and the initiation of therapeutic action that will follow. This connection stems, at least in part, from the beneficial impact that the latter can have on the former. The various ill effects associated with obesity, for example, may result from excessive food intake as well as insufficient physical activity. The therapeutic use of exercise—along with changes in dietary habits, of course—has therefore become a widely used tool in the alleviation of obesity problems.

In general, obesity is a condition of excess adipose tissue relative to lean body mass that currently is defined as body weight greater than 20% of standard for height and frame size. The problem today is considered a widespread nutritional disorder that predisposes the individual who suffers from it to a shortened life span and an increased chance of developing heart disease, diabetes, and cancer.

Excess weight also can adversely affect an individual's self-image, and oftentimes it even will have a negative impact on his or her status in the community. Because of its many ramifications, it is crucial for the clinician to be able to determine the degree of obesity—and the reasons behind it—in order to regulate treatment.

In many cases, psychological factors play an important role in the development of obesity. The clinician must take a thorough and accurate case history in order to isolate the precise factors contributing to the problem before successful treatment can begin. Of primary concern are genetics, the environment, food intake, and exercise habits.

Throughout the process, the practitioner always should remember that a patient's body weight is determined by his or her ability to balance energy intake and energy expediture. If the expenditure is increased while the intake remains constant, the patient's weight will naturally decrease. Often, such a strategy is easier for patients to follow than one dependent solely upon dietary restrictions. In addition to weight loss, it also will have an impact on the patient's body composition and metabolic rate.

Special Considerations: Case History

Duration of obesity
Sudden or gradual onset of weight
Juvenile or adult onset of obesity
Family history of obesity
Level of exercise
Psychological factors:
  Does the patient:
    Eat more under stress?
    Eat while watching television?
    Eat while preparing meals?
    Eat while reading or studying?
    Overeat primarily when alone?
    Use food as a reward?
    Have low self-esteem?
  Is the patient:
    A night eater
    Binge eater
    Nibbler
    Smoker
    Drinker
Lower socioeconomic status
Recent change(s) in personal life
Are any of the following associated diseases present:
  Diabetes
  Hypoglycemia
  Arthritis
  Coronary artery disease
  Atherosclerosis
  High blood pressure
  Hypertriglyceridemia
  Hypercholesterolemia
  Hypoventilation

Special Considerations: Dietary History

Portion sizes
Food cravings
Food choices

Energy-dense foods
Gravies, sauces
Food preparation habits
Does the patient regularly:
Fry
Sauté
Use butter or margerine as flavoring

Special Considerations: Physical Examination

The patient must be examined carefully to determine the extent of obesity as well as for any signs of malnutrition. Even though the patient is overweight, there may be multiple vitamin and mineral deficiencies caused by a poor diet. See Chapter 1 for causes of vitamin and mineral deficiencies and for physical signs of suboptimnal nutrition.

Special Considerations: Anthropometric Measurements

Check weight/height
Skin fold thickness:
Triceps subscapular
Lower abdomen
Thigh
Arm circumference
Arm muscle circumference
Arm muscle area
Body type:
Ectomorph
Endomorph

Special Considerations: Drug-Nutrient Interactions

Many patients who are overweight use medications to control obesity and related diseases.
The clinician must obtain a complete drug history including:

Drugs presently taken
Previous drugs
Self-administered medications

Some drugs to be aware of in relation to the obese include:

Diuretics
Amphetamines
Oral diabetic agents
Insulin
Cardiac glycosides
Thyroid medication

Drug-related obesities include:

Cyproheptadine
Phenothiazines
Tricyclic antidepressants

Special Considerations: Laboratory Examination

Endocrine disorders:

Hypothyroidism

Hypopituitarism
Insulinoma
Reactive hypoglycemia
Thyroid deficiency

Anorexia Nervosa

Eating disorders are deviations in a patient's pattern of dietary intake that can lead to disease. They may result in extreme fatness or extreme thinness. The assessment of conditions leading to the former is discussed earlier in this chapter under the heading "Obesity"; a nutritional assessment for behavior that leads to the latter is detailed below.

Of the several eating disorders that can cause a patient to become extremely thin, anorexia nervosa has received perhaps the most attention in recent years. It is a complex condition that arises from a refusal to eat. It develops when a patient becomes abnormally concerned with obtaining a low body weight, and it can lead to severe weight loss, emaciation, and occasionally death.

Typically, the anorexic is a young woman—there is a 12:1 female:male ratio among those who suffer from the disorder—and victims often had been overweight earlier in adolescence. Typically, it also develops among those who belong to the middle class and come from apparently stable family situations. Some unresolved food-related conflict usually exists, however, which may be aggravated by our society's current connection between thinness and physical beauty.

Anorexics develop strange patterns of dietary intake and their thoughts about food often are bizarre and all-consuming. Many, for example, are able to repress the sensation of hunger while constantly thinking about food. They may exercise constantly while using laxatives or diuretics and vomiting voluntarily. They may have a distorted body image that leads them to believe they are overweight when in fact they actually are underweight. The resultant behavior may lead to a body weight loss of 25% or more, and, ultimately, to starvation.

The clinician dealing with an anorexic must assess the degree of weight loss and of lean muscle mass in order to determine the form of treatment. In severe cases, psychiatric treatment and/or hospitalization will be required.

Special Considerations: Case History

Onset of symptoms
Was the patient overweight before becoming anorexic?
Was he or she teased about weight?
Frequent or prolonged periods of physical exercise?
Does the patient:
  Gorge
  Vomit
Does the patient use:
  Laxatives
  Diuretics
  Tranquilizers
  Antidepressants
Is the patient hyperactive?
Is amenorrhea present?
Is the patient obsessed with food?
Psychological factors:
  Is there conflict within family—especially between the female teenage anorexic and her parents?

Has food been used as a punishment?
Has food been used as a reward?
Is the female anorexic refusing to accept her sexual identity?

Special Considerations: Dietary History

Severely restricted food intake
Self-induced vomiting

Special Considerations: Physical Examination

Deficiency states must be monitored carefully as the patient often has multiple vitamin and mineral deficiencies. The physical examination should be thorough as the clinician checks for the deficiency symptoms detailed in Chapter 1. In addition, the patient should be checked for:

Fluid and electrolyte imbalances
Hypokalemia
Hypogeusia
Dysgeusia
Alopecia
Overhydration that can lead to pulmonary edema and death
Dehydration from:
    Laxatives
    Diuretics
    Antidepressants
Loss of dental substance
Poor skin turgor
Weakness
Parotid salivary gland enlargement
Esophagitis
Upper gastrointestinal bleeding (Mallory-Weiss tears)
Hoarseness or sore throat
Anal irritation
Thinning hair
Changes in hair texture

Special Considerations: Anthropometric Measurements

All anthropometric tests should be carefully assessed to determine the extent and pattern of weight loss and the degree of protein-calorie malnutrition. (See Tables 3.1–3.5 for more information.)

Special Considerations: Laboratory Examination

Serum albumin
Transferrin
Prealbumin
Lymphocyte count
Serum Zn
Serum Cu
Signs of frequent or prolonged vomiting:
    Reduced serum K
    Reduced serum Cl
    Stools turning red upon addition of NaOH

Athletic Performance

The basis of athletic performance often is considered to be primarily nutritional. To varying degrees, this applies to the professional athlete in addition to the participant in weekend sporting events. Therefore, a patient's nutritional status usually will have a tremendous bearing upon his or her physical abilities while the engagement of these abilities will likewise have a noticeable impact on nutritional status. Any clinical assessment during these times of heightened physical fitness activity, then, must naturally include an examination of these specific causes and effects.

Even the most casual observer or sedentary cynic today would be hard-pressed to deny that physical activity changes body composition—and usually for the better. Those who exercise are more likely to remain healthy than those who do not. They have strengthened hearts, lungs, and circulatory systems, as well as an easier time maintaining their optimal body weight. In addition, regular physical activity also increases the ability of their muscle fibers to produce energy and the ability of their hormones to regulate energy metabolism.

In order to accurately assess the athletic patient, the clinician must examine food intake and dietary patterns specifically as they relate to the release of energy. The under- or overconsumption of carbohydrates, fats, and proteins, for example, may have a significant impact on a patient's athletic performance. At the same time, excessive or deficient ingestion of vitamins and minerals also may affect the patient's ability to reach peak performance levels.

Additionally, the physically active patient will record anthropometric and body composition levels that often are quite different from those considered to be "normal." It therefore is important for the practitioner to recognize these patients quickly and remember to judge them on standards that more closely match their own population averages.

Special Considerations: Case History

Children, adolescents, and pregnant women require additional attention.
Exercise-induced asthma is possible.
Female patients may report amenorrhea or oligomenorrhea.
Risks to hypertensive patients can be increased by isometric, free weight and hydraulic exercise.

Special Considerations: Dietary History

Does patient:
Eat breakfast regularly?
Consume adequate calcium (especially women)?
Avoid fats?
Use steroids?
Consume adequate water, particularly during sporting events?
Diet regularly to achieve and maintain optimal weight?
Incidence of iron deficiency is higher than in other populations (especially among younger athletes).
Increased caloric consumption is necessary.
Possible increased need for protein.
Increased need for thiamine, riboflavin, and niacin.
Increased need for carbohydrates.
Possible increased need for certain B vitamins.

Special Considerations: Physical Examination

Delayed growth and development are possible in younger athletes. The following features may be related:

Pallor

Edema

Thinning hair

Changes in hair texture

Systolic and diastolic blood pressure may be lowered through aerobic exercise.

Renal blood flow is reduced by exercise.

Resting and submaximal heart rate will be lower than for sedentary population.

Maximal cardiac output will be increased by exercise.

Palpation of the cartoid artery is the accepted means of determining actual heart rate during and immediately after exercise.

Special Considerations: Anthropometric Measurements

Standard height-weight tables may be inappropriate.

Body fat standards are different for active individuals:

Athletes: 12 to 15% men, 20 to 25% women

Top athletes: 7 to 10% men, 12 to 18% women

Ideal lean body weight varies according to athletic pursuit.

Special Considerations: Laboratory Testing

Hemoglobin concentrations may be in low- to midrange of the population norms.

Sustained vigorous exercise may increase the metabolic rate 20 to 25 times.

Check for lowered levels of:

Serum albumin

Transferrin

Prealbumin

Lymphocyte count

Exercise can increase these hormone secretions:

Growth hormone

Thyrotopin

Prolactin

Endomorphins

Vasopressin

Cortisol

Corticosterone

Aldosterone

Epinephrine

Norepinephrine

Thyroxine T4

Triiodothyronine T3

Insulin

Glucagon

Estrogen

Progesterone

Testosterone

Renin

Musculoskeletal System

Patients who suffer from diseases of the musculoskeletal system usually experience altered nutritional status because of the impact on their dietary intake patterns. Arthritis, for one common example, may make it too painful for proper food preparation to commence and for regular eating patterns to be continued. Additionally, dental caries and periodontal disease may lead to the exclusion of certain foods that are difficult to chew but necessary for complete nutrition.

Poor nutritional status, on the other hand, also can lead to musculoskeletal diseases. Osteoporosis is one related condition affecting women over the course of many years that has received much attention in recent years in both the professional and the lay press. The development of various dental problems also may result from improper food intake.

Nutrition-related factors that are particularly important to watch during the assessment of patients with diseases of the musculoskeletal system are their use of drugs and their consumption of certain foods. The status of a patient's teeth, bowel and bladder control, and physical movement also may be relevant in this area.

Special Considerations: Case History

Does the patient find food preparation difficult?
Is eating or chewing painful?
Does the patient consume large quantities of:
  Aspirin
  Aluminum-containing antacids
Are there complaints about:
  Skeletal pain
  Muscle weakness
Is the patient physically active?
Have "fad diets" been employed?
Is there a family hisotry of osteoporosis?

Special Considerations: Dietary History

High phosphate intake
High fat intake
High carbohydrate intake
Consumption of foods with high purine content
Alcohol abuse (especially beer)
High sucrose consumption
Frequent snacking
Low protein consumption
Low calcium consumption
Adequate intake of zinc and vitamins C and E

Special Considerations: Physical Examination

Arthritis (rheumatoid or atrophic)
Dental caries
Periodontal disease
Poorly fitting dentures
Osteoporosis
Osteomalacia
Gastrointestinal disorders
Fractures
Leg bowing
Stooped posture
Unsteady gait

Movement problems
Decreased height
Edema in muscles, joints, bones
Fever, leading to:
    Anorexia
    Weight loss
    Inanition (in severe cases)

Special Considerations: Drug-Nutrient Interaction

Does the patient take:
    Isoniazid
    Corticosteroids
    Tetracycline
    Thyroid preparations
    Furosemide
    Heparin
    Antiinflammatory agents
        Indomethacin (Indocin)
        Phenylbutazone
        Sulindac (Clinoril)
        Ibuprofin
    Steroids

Special Considerations: Laboratory Testing

Estrogen deficiency
Negative nitrogen balance

Food Allergies

The term "food allergy," when used in the most general sense, has come to refer to an abnormal response to any food that usually is tolerated by the population at large. If such an overly broad definition is used, however, the clinician may have a tendency to overdiagnose this problem and then fail to spot and treat the actual illness from which an apparent symptom really stems. A more narrow definition, on the other hand, relates food allergies only to those conditions resulting in an anaphylactic response. However, this approach can lead to underdiagnosis and then to the inadequate treatment of a true food allergy.

In order to alleviate these potential problems, in recent years a clinically significant food allergy has come to mean any adverse reaction to food involving an immune mechanism. Other terms now generally used by clinicians to describe related conditions include food intolerance (an abnormal physiological response to an ingested food component or additive), food toxicity (an adverse reaction caused by direct action of food that may involve nonimmune release of chemical mediators), and food idiosyncrasy (a disproportionate response to food that is unrelated to any physiological, pharmacological or immune effects).

Documented physical symptoms of food allergies may develop in the gastrointestinal tract, respiratory tract, or the skin. Such responses may range from mild to severe, and even include respiratory failure and death. Additionally, psychological and behavioral symptoms also have been pinpointed by certain practioners. These responses—considered unproven by others—remain a source of controversy; they include hyperactivity, fatigue, lethargy, aches, pains, and learning disabilities.

Nonetheless, the detection of true food allergies during a patient's assessment is an important step in the determination of nutritional status. And it certainly is critical to the eventual management of the resultant problems. Such identification also may be particularly important in young children, when food allergies can lead to growth failure.

Special Considerations: Case History

Does the patient report:
Mental confusion
Depression
Migraine headaches
Diarrhea
Vomiting
Abdominal pain
Abdominal distention
Flatulence
Constipation
Bloating
Asthma
Dizziness
Blurred vision
Gastrointestinal disorders
Chronic ear infections
Recurrent croup
Postnasal discharge
Numbness of extremities
Paralysis
What are the frequency and duration of such reactions?
Is there any evidence of allergic tension fatigue syndromes (ATFSs):
Hyperactivity
Fatigue
Lethargy
Aches of muscles or joints
Behavioral learning disorders
Is there any family history of food allergies?

Special Considerations: Dietary History

What foods were consumed within 72 hours of any reactions reported above?
How much of that food was consumed?
Have any new foods been introduced to the patient's diet?

Special Considerations: Physical Examination

Check for the presence of:
Allergic dermatitis
Contact dermatitis
Anaphylaxis
Angioedema
Pruritus
Rashes
Rhinitis
Urticaria

Edema
Eczema
Entereopathies
Malabsorption
Gross bleeding
Occult bleeding
Pneumonitis
Hypoglycemia
Are there dark circles under the patient's eyes (allergic shiners)?

Special Considerations: Laboratory Testing

Inhibited protein synthesis
Elevated serum phenylalanine levels
Evidence of:
  Anemia
  Eosinophilia
  Thrombocytopenia

Anemias

Nutritional anemia is defined as a condition in which the patient suffers from a deficiency in the size or the number of red blood cells (erythrocytes), or in which the hemoglobin concentration is below the level that is normal for a given individual. Because blood is the body's main transportation system for nutrients, the existence of anemia will have a strong impact on the patient's nutritional status.

The presence of anemia results from a deficiency of one or more of the nutrients required for hemopoiesis. Those of greatest importance are iron (the most commonly deficient nutrient in the world), Vitamin B$_{12}$, and folic acid. Additionally, deficiencies in protein, pyridoxine, ascorbic acid, copper and other heavy metals also may lead to anmeia, as can an infestation of the gastrointestinal tract by parasitic worms that feed on blood (bloodworm) or on nutrients (tapeworm).

The clinician who is assessing an anemic patient should look for the cause of such a deficiency; these can include inadequate intake, improper absorption, imperfect utilization, injury to the bone marrow, or increased requirements (such as those stemming from pregnancy or adolescence). Any of these can lead to the depletion of nutritional stores and eventually result in anemia.

Special Considerations: Case History

Does the patient have concurrent illness or disease:
  Asthma
  Cancer
  Cardiovascular disease
  Hemorrhage
  Myocardial infarction
  Renal disease
Has there been surgery, especially:
  Gastric
  Hepatic
  Renal
Has the patient had infections, sepsis?

Is there a family history of:
Allergies
Anemias
Cancer
Leukemias
Immune disorders
Does the patient use:
Alcohol
Nicotine
Does the patient suffer from anorexia?
Does the patient suffer from fatigue?

Special Considerations: Dietary History

What are the patient's habits regarding intake of heme versus nonheme iron? Decreased protein intake?

Special Considerations: Physical Examination

Beefy, red tongue

Special Considerations: Laboratory Testing

There are several tests that the clinician can use for the evaluation of iron status. Listed along with their various advantages and disadvantages, they include:

1. Hemoglobin
   Advantages:
   Widely available
   Inexpensive
   Fairly rapid results
   Disadvantages:
   Not specific
   Relatively insensitive
2. Serum iron and iron-binding capacity
   Advantages:
   Widely available
   Moderate cost
   Fairly specific
   Disadvantages:
   Moderate sensitivity
   Diurnal variation (iron)
   Time-consuming methodology
   Extraneous iron contamination
   Drugs influence results
   Does not reflect amount of stored iron
   Results influenced by inflammatory conditions, malignancy and acute infection
3. Percentage of saturation of transferrin
   This is the ratio of serum-iron concentration to total iron-binding capacity expressed as a percentage. A value of 16% or lower indicates lack of iron stores.
   Advantages:
   Widely available

Simple to determine
Inexpensive
Sensitive test
Disadvantages:
Time-consuming method
Subject to error from extraneous iron contamination
Precision limited by diurnal variations
Results influenced by mild or transient infection

4. Serum transferrin
Serum transferrin is the iron-transporting protein produced by the liver.
Advantages:
Direct measurement
Precision greater than chemical methods for total iron-binding capacity (TIBC)
Disadvantages:
Not widely available
Offers no real advantages over existing methods for TIBC
Influenced by malignancy, chronic disorders, liver disease and drugs

5. Free erythrocyte protoporphyrin
Protoporphyrin is the complex that combines with iron to form hemoglobin. A limitation in iron supply to red cell precursors is reflected by an increase in unbound protoporphyyrin of circulating red cells.
Advantages:
Relatively greater stability than transferrin saturation
Specific, precise
Disadvantages:
Not widely available
Less sensitive than other techniques in detecting mild degrees of iron deficiency

6. Serum ferritin
The major iron storage protein in the body, serum ferritin detoxifies cellular iron and recycles it for hematopoiesis. Serum concentration reflects iron stores.
Advantages:
Sensitive and precise test that gives an accurate picture of iron stores
Useful in distinguishing iron deficiency from anemia or chronic disease
Disadvantages:
Moderately expensive
Serum levels influenced by hemolytic, inflammatory, neoplastic, and hepatic disorders
Not useful during or immediately after oral iron therapy

Laboratory Tests for Evaluation of Folate Status

Serum Folate
Red blood cell (RBC) Folate
Formiminogolutamic acid (FIGLU)
Deoxyuridine suppression test
Description of Deoxyuridine Suppression Test
Aid to diagnosis in difficult cases
Depends upon two ALT pathways for synthesis of the nucleotide thymidylic acid—DNA
Folic acid necessary
Performed: peripheral blood lymphocytes phytohemagglutinin stimulation

Previously treated megaloblastic anemia
Interpretation of Serum and Red Cell Folate Results

Comparison of Microbiological and Radioisotopic Methods

The morphological changes in the peripheral blood and bone marrow due to folate deficiency are identical to those of Vitamin B$_{12}$ deficiency. To determine the difference, an assay of the two vitamins must be done. Folate deficiency occurs in a wide variety of clinical conditions such as alcoholism, malnutrition, malabsorption, renal dialysis, and patients taking anticonvulsive drugs. It also appears in conditions with increased utilization including pregnancy, hemolytic anemia, and malignancy. Folate deficiency also may contribute to fetal abnormalities and possibly neurological disease with no anemia and few, if any, changes in the peripheral blood.

Red cell folate is an index of tissue folate concentrations, whereas serum folate is concerned as much with transport and exchange of folate between body compartments as with nutritional status.

The radioassay offers several advantages over the microbiological method, particularly in that it is not affected by antibiotics or antimetabolites and can be performed by any laboratory with a gamma counter.

Red blood cell folate determinations are a reflection of tissue levels of folate. Low serum levels may only reflect recent low dietary intakes of the vitamin and provide little information concerning tissue reserves.

Formiminoglutamic Acid (FIGLU)

Several indirect tests for evaluating folacin status are based on the increased urinary excretion of FIGLU and of its immediate precursor urocanic acid, which occurs in the folacin-deficient subject. The excretion of FIGLU and/or of FIGLU plus urocanic acid has been a useful index of folate deficiency, particularly in research studies. However, for nutritional assessment, the procedure is impractical. The abnormal excretion of the metabolites appears to correlate better with red cell folates than with serum folates.

Interpretation and Application of Serum Folate Levels

Increased:
  Intestinal blind-loop syndrome
  Vitamin B$_{12}$ deficiency (found in ⅓ of patients)
  Certain congenital enzyme deficiencies
Decreased:
  Inadequate intake:
    Alcoholism
    Improper cooking
    Food faddism
    Poverty
  Defective utilization:
    Liver disease
    Megaloblastic anemia
  Malabsorption:
    Sprue
    Celiac disease
    Idiopathic steatorrhea
    Blind-loop syndrome

Crohn's regional ileitis
Intestinal resection
Tubercular enteritis
Lymphoma affecting small intestine
Interference with folic acid activity
Folic acid antagonists:
Cytotoxic drugs
Ethyl alcohol
Pyrimethamine
Anticonvulsants
Excessive utilization due to marked cellular proliferation:
Hemolytic anemias
Myeloproliferative disorders
Carcinomas
Enzyme deficiency (homocystinuria)
Rheumatoid arthritis
Low birth weight
Long term renal dialysis
Malnutrition and chronic infections in infants

Laboratory Tests for Evaluation of Vitamin B_{12} Status

1. Serum B_{12} Assay

    The principle of the test is that serum is added as a source of vitamin B_{12} to a medium containing all essential growth factors for vitamin B_{12} dependent microorganisms. The medium is then inoculated with the microorganism and the amount of B_{12} is then inoculated in the serum. A determination is made by comparing the growth as estimated turbimetrically with the growth produced by a standard amount of Vitamin B_{12}. The two microorganisms used for B_{12} assay are *Euglena gracilis* and *Lactobacilus leichmannii*. The microbiological assay is lengthy and shows interference by various drugs (antibiotics and antimetabolites) that inhibit growth and could produce artificially low results.

2. Radioassay

    This technique is rapid and shows minimal interference relative to the microbiological assay. Some reports of large doses of ascorbic acid (2 gm per day) or in vitro fluoride (as a preservative) may interfere in the B_{12} radioassay. More extensive use of this assay has revealed technical problems that result in higher values for serum cobalamin than the value. In fact an estimated 20% of patients with B_{12} deficiency may have been misdiagnosed as having normal B_{12} levels with the radioassay procedure. On the average only 20% of the binders in commercial radioassay kits consist of extrinsic factor. The remainder consists of a protein referred to as R protein that binds with biologically inactive cobalamin as well as in true human plasma. New kits appear to have resolved this problem through the use of an agent that blocks the nonspecific binding by R proteins.

3. RBC B_{12} assay

    Measurement of erythrocyte B_{12} content is of less value in the diagnosis of vitamin B_{12} deficiency than serum determinations. The RBC B_{12} assay may be more useful in estimated tissue stores than is serum when the serum levels are artificially elevated (i.e., in liver disease, recent B_{12} injections, and chronic myelogenous leukemia).

4. Urinary excretion of methylmalonic acid

   Vitamin B_{12} deficiency is associated with an increase of methylmalonic acid excretion in the urine as the isomerization of methylmalonyl-CoA requires the vitamin B_{12} coenzyme. Concurrent oral administration of valine or isoleucine further increases the amount excreted. At the present time a simple and satisfactory technique for measuring urinary excretion is not available and the present test lacks diagnostic precision.

5. Radioactive B_{12} absorption test (Schilling test)

   This test is used to measure vitamin B_{12} absorption. A small amount of radioactive B_{12} is given orally followed by a large nonradioactive dose of vitamin B_{12} (given parenterally). The urine is collected for 24 and 48 hours. If the radioactive oral B_{12} is absorbed the large dose of parenterally administered nonradioactive B_{12} will flush significant amounts of radioactive B_{12} into the urine. If the test results are abnormal, the test may be repeated giving the intrinsic factor with the radioactive oral dose.

   Normal subjects will excrete more than 7% of the administered radioactive B_{12} in a 24-hour urine collection. Patients with pernicious anemia will usually excrete less than 3%. When the intrinsic factor is added, excretion rises to the normal range. Falsely low values may result from acute renal disease, which impairs urinary excretion of vitamin B_{12}.

Schilling Test Results

Cause: Prolonged inadequate intake of B_{12}
Without Intrinsic Factor: Normal
With Intrinsic Factor: Normal

Cause: Absence of intrinsic factor (pernicious anemia)
Without Intrinsic Factor: Abnormal
With Intrinsic Factor: Normal

Cause: Small bowel disease—Malabsorption
Without Intrinsic Factor: Abnormal
With Intrinsic Factor: Abnormal

Cause: Bacterial competition for B_{12}
Without Intrinsic Factor: Abnormal
With Intrinsic Factor: Abnormal

Immune System

Prolonged malnutrition will have a severe effect on a variety of systems in the human body. One of the most important to the practitioner who is assessing nutritional status is the potential impact that such a condition will have on a patient's immune responses. These often are particularly extreme when a deficiency is aggravated by the presence of an infection, which then can lead to an increased metabolic rate or catabolism.

The clinician undertaking a nutritional assessment should note that immunodeficiencies often result from the deficiency of several nutrients, particularly when an infection also exists. These nutrients include amino acids, zinc, copper, magnesium, selenium, vitamins B_6, C, A, and B_{12}, folic acid, pantothenic acid, riboflavin.

In conjunction with a deficiency in any of these nutrients, the patient's immune responses can be suppressed by a number of factors. Those for which the clinician should check include:

1. The disruption of mucosal and cutaneous integrity
2. The depression of cell-mediated immunity
3. The impairment of humoral antibody production
4. The diminishment of nonspecific resistance factors.
5. The reduction of phagocytic activity.
6. The retarding of wound healing.

Nutrition and Mucocutaneous Integrity

Vitamin A deficiency
>The specialized epithelium lining of the respiratory and urinary tracts, eyes, glands, and hair follicles undergo metaplastic conversion into keratinizing, stratified, squamous epithelium. Infections are then more likely to develop.

Niacin deficiency
>Dermatitis develops
>Mucositis
>Patient more likely to develop secondary infections, including ulceronecrotizing Vincent's infection.
>Riboflavin deficiency
>Can develop macerated angles of mouth that become infected by organisms introduced via tongue licking.

Folic acid and vitamin B_{12} deficiency
>Megaloblastic changes take place in the actively replicating tissues (i.e., in bone marrow and oral mucosa).
>The ulcerated mucositis is highly conducive to superimposed infection.

Pyridoxine deficiency
>Impairs nucleic acid synthesis
>Where dermatitis is present, there is a strong tendency to develop infections.

Vitamin C deficiency
>Intense gingival reddening
>Scorbutic gingivitis
>Prone to secondary infections
>Iron deficiency
>Widespread tissue defects including normoblastic arrest in bone marrow to microcytosis in the oral epithelium.
>In iron deficiency anemia, the atrophic glossitis and angular cheilosis predispose to local infections especially by *Candida albicans*.

Nutrition and Cell-Mediated Immunity

Cell-mediated immunity plays an important role in defending against viral, microbacterial, and protozoal and fungal infections. The clinician should watch for:

Protein-calorie malnutrition
>In children with kwashiorkor, marasmus, and mixed marasmus-kwashiorkor and in debilitated hospital patients, there is a depressed cell-mediated immune function that is shown by:
>Lymphopenia
>Low T-cell number in circulating blood
>Diminished tonsil size
>Decreased reactivity to delayed skin test antigens (tuberculin, *Candida*, trichophyton, diptheria toxoid, streptokinase-streptodornase).

Iron deficiency
Impairs lymphocyte transformation
Pyridoxine deficiency
Severe thymic atrophy
Lymphocyte depression
Zinc deficiency
Thymic atrophy in children with protein-calorie malnutrition
Depressed cell-mediated immunity
Nutrition and Humoral Antibody Production
Secretory IgA (contributes to resistance to infection along mucosal surface)
Deficiency of pyridoxine, folic acid, pantothenic acid, thiamine, biotin, riboflavin, niacin, tryptophan, pro-vitamin A, and vitamin C inhibit antibody formation.
Pantothenic acid deficiency
Poor response to tetanus antigen
Pyridoxine deficiency
Reduced reaction to tetanus, typhoid O and H antigens
Suppressed capacity to mount antibodies to tetanus and typhoid antigen when there is a combined pantothenic acid-pyridoxine deficiency.
Children with protein-calorie malnutrition
Secretory IgA in salivary, nasopharyngeal, and lacrimal secretions is significantly decreased, which contributes to increased proneness to mucocutaneous infections.

Nutrition and Nonspecific Resistance Factors

The complement system
Children with protein-calorie malnutrition have a significant decrease in total hemolytic complement activity and the level of almost all components except C4. This is most pronounced when infection is present.
Lysozyme
In the serum, tears, saliva, sweat, respiratory and intestinal mucus, neutrophils, and monocytes there is a decrease in lysozyme activity, especially in malnourished children. Mucosal and glandular lysozyme activity is markedly diminished or abolished in patients with a vitamin A deficiency.
Properdin
A serum euglobulin associated with nonspecific natural resistance to infections of bacterial, viral, and protozoal origin.
Interferon
Supplements other mechanisms of resistance to viral and other infections. Interferon may be depressed in nutritional deficiencies that interfere with protein production.
Transferrin and lactoferrin
These iron-binding proteins have innate bacteriocide and bacteriostatic properties. They are decreased in protein-calorie malnutrition, especially kwashiorkor, and are adversely affected by deficiency states that diminish protein production.

Nutrition and Phagocytosis

Iron deficiency
Depresses activity of enzymes necessary for distribution of phagocytized microorganisms.
Folic acid deficiency

Can cause leukopenia, granulocytopenia, macrocytic anemia, and thrombo-cytopenia.

Nutrition and Wound Healing

Zinc deficiency
Associated with impairment of host defenses and tissue repair.
Ascorbic acid deficiency
Prevents the formation of collagen molecules.
Protein, ascorbic acid, zinc deficiencies
Retards wound healing and repair of infected lesions.

Cardiovascular Disease

In recent years, increasing attention has been paid to cardiovascular disease by clinicians and patients alike. Nonetheless, it remains a very serious problem in the United States and still is responsible for as many as half of all of the deaths in the nation each year. Coronary disease and stroke account for about 75% of this total, and so any assessment of nutritional status should focus heavily on the risk factors that can lead to these ailments.

More and more, cardiovascular disease is thought to be related to lifestyle choices—many of which can be modified once they are identified. The type of food that a patient consumes, for example, may have the largest impact on his or her potential for contracting cardiovascular disease. Exercise, stress, alcohol use, and tobacco smoking also have been identified as risk factors that can be eliminated. Those that also may play a part in the development of the disease but are not possible to control include the patient's age, sex, and family history.

Because the presence of high levels of serum cholesterol is largely responsible for the prevalence of cardiovascular disease in contemporary society, it often is considered to be the area that should be checked most closely by the clinician. Others to examine carefully include the ingestion of salt and saturated fatty acids, the presence of hypertension or obesity, and the amount and quality of exercise that the patient reports.

Special Considerations: Case History

Is the patient:
Male
Woman after menopause
Over 40
Is there a family history of:
Hyperlipidemia
Hypertension
Coronary artery disease (especially before age 55)
Does the patient smoke cigarettes?
Does the patient report:
Diabetes mellitus
A sedentary lifestyle
A stressful lifestyle
Chest pains
Does the patient exhibit type A behavior?

Special Considerations: Dietary History

Daily use of foods high in saturated fat and cholesterol
Daily use of high-sodium foods and salt at the table
Relative lack of dietary fiber-rich foods

Excess energy intake
Does the patient consume:
  Egg yolks
  Whole milk
  Ice cream
  Whole milk yogurt
  Cheese
  Butter
  Fried foods
  Commercial baked goods
  Egg noodles
  Fatty meats (pork, beef, lamb)
  Sausage
  Organ meats
  Hot dogs
  Bacon
  Bacon fat
  Lard
  Fruits, vegetables in cream sauce, or butter
  "Junk food" snacks
  Instant beverage drinks
  Eggnog
  Coconut, palm, or palm kernel oils
  Hydrogenated vegetable oils
  Coffee
  Vegetable salts and flakes
  Smoked, processed, or cured meats and fish
  Salad dressings containing cheese
  Macadamia nuts or cashews
  Mayonnaise or margarine with unidentified vegetable oil on the label

Special Considerations: Physical Examination

Patient is severely overweight (more than 120% of ideal)
Presence of xanthomas, or yellowish plaques deposited on skin (rare)
Edema, ascites
Elevated blood pressure

Special Considerations: Anthropometric Measurements

Skinfold measurements in 95th percentile for age and sex.

Special Considerations: Laboratory Testing

Because the close connection between serum cholesterol and cardiovascular disease has been made, it is critical that all patients undergo appropriate laboratory measurements. High density lipoproteins (HDLs) can be assessed in most clinical laboratories; low density lipoproteins (LDLs) can be calculated if the patient's triglyceride level is less than 400 mg/dl by the following formula:
Triglycerides

$$LDL = \text{Serum Cholesterol} - HDL - \frac{\text{Triglycerides}}{5}$$

Risk ratios are outlined in Table 6.1; specific information on HDL and LDL cholesterol and lipid abnormality investigation follows.

Table 6.1.
Cholesterol Risk Ratios
The chart illustrates a method for determining risk ratios for LDL cholesterol, or total cholesterol and HDL cholesterol, for both men and women.

	LDL Cholesterol ÷ HDL Cholesterol	Total Cholesterol ÷ HDL Cholesterol
Risk in Men		
½ Average	1.00	3.43
Average	3.55	4.97
2 × Average	6.25	9.55
3 × Average	7.99	23.39
Risk in Women		
½ Average	1.47	3.27
Average	3.22	4.44
2 × Average	5.03	7.05
3 × Average	6.14	11.04

High Density Lipoproteins (HDLs)

There is little known about the function of HDL, but it appears to be a reservoir for apoprotein C2 and a scavenger for lipids during lipolysis. It also may play a role in triglyceride metabolism. Low levels of HDL are consistent with a higher risk of coronary heart disease. In particular, HDL2 seems to play a significant role in decreased coronary problems. Higher levels of HDL appear to be protective in the prevention of coronary heart disease.

Lower levels are associated with:

Male sex

Oral contraceptives

Obesity

Poor diabetes control

Cigarette smoking

Higher levels are associated with:

Female sex

Exercise

Moderate alcohol consumption

Vegetarian diet

Complex carbohydrate consumption

Low Density Lipoproteins (LDLs)

LDLs appear to be elevated in those individuals who are at risk for coronary heart disease. The LDLs are composed of nearly half cholesterol with equal amounts of triglycerides and phospholipids and approximately 20% protein.

An approach to the investigation of lipid abnormalities

A patient who is considered at risk for coronary heart disease should have an evaluation of his lipid status. Patient preparation includes maintenance of their usual diet and a fast for a minimum of 10 hours before the laboratory tests. The following should be ordered to calculate the risk ratios:

Serum cholesterol

Triglycerides

HDL cholesterol

LDL cholesterol

Geriatrics and Degenerative Disease

People over age 65 comprise a growing percentage of the population of the United States. They also have a variety of physical and economic problems that could lead to a less than satisfactory nutritional status. These include a lack of teeth, decreased salivation and absorption capabilities, diminished senses of taste and smell, lowered income levels, and increased use of prescription and over-the-counter drugs.

In addition, a number of degenerative diseases are more apt to strike older Americans than those of any other age group. Like age itself, these diseases often present their own obstacles to the attainment of optimal nutritional status.

Because of the size of these two affected groups—and the fact that their members use the greatest portion of our health care resources—the challenge facing clinicians attempting to assess the nutritional status of geriatrics and those with degenerative disease is great. The practitioner, therefore, must remember that patients in these categories are more likely to have nutritional deficiencies and then assess them with the help of a very thorough case history and physical examination that specifically address their special needs and requirements.

Special Considerations: Case History

In addition to the questions raised in Chapter 1, the clinician must be careful to determine:

If symptoms of disease or illness exists, how long have they been present?
Is there a familial history of the same disease?
Has the patient been hospitalized for this condition?
Have symptoms ever regressed?
    If so, under what conditions?
Is the patient on any drugs?
    If so, for how long?
Does the patient live alone?
Does the patient eat alone?
Are there adequate facilities for:
    Cooking
    Food storage
Is the patient strong enough to cook for him/herself?
Is there adequate income for a balanced diet?
Is the patient able to shop for groceries?
Does the patient have problems with:
    Gas
    Constipation
    Poor digestion
    Inability to chew
    Bloating
    Cramping
    Lactose intolerance
    Diarrhea after milk consumption
    Vision impairment
Does the patient have poorly fitting dentures?
Is the patient overweight?
    For how long?
Is the patient underweight?
    For how long?

Has there been a recent, rapid weight loss?
Has there been decreased physical activity with:
   Retirement
   Chronic disease
Has there been recent loss of the patient's spouse?
Are there family members and friends nearby?
Does the patient drink alcohol?
Has the patient suffered an altered mental state?
Is the patient lethargic?

Special Considerations: Dietary History

Unpalatable therapeutic diet
Decreased intake of high fiber foods
Inadequate intake of vitamin D-fortified milk products
Decreased intake of animal protein

Special Considerations: Physical Examination

The high risk factor of nutritional deficiencies makes the physical examination of utmost importance. The clinician must check carefully for any nutritional deficiencies while watching for:

Muscle wasting
Edema
Thinning of hair
Changes in hair texture
Poor skin turgor
Dry, sticky muscous membranes
Any of the following conditions:
   Hypogeusia
   Dysgeusia
   Alopecia
   Dermatitis

Special Considerations: Anthropometric Measurement

The patient should be checked both for obesity and protein-calorie malnutrition as described in Chapter 3. Particular attention must be paid to:

Body weight
Body fat
Height loss

Special Considerations: Laboratory Testing

Evidence of protein-calorie malnutrition, inadequate fluid balance, and inadequate mineral intake may be uncovered through analysis of:

Serum albumin
Transferrin
Prealbumin
Lymphocyte count
Nonreactive skin tests
Hematological measures

Hemoglobin
Hematocrit
Mean serum iron
Total iron-binding capacity
Blood urea nitrogen
Serum zinc

Hospitalized Patient

Recent studies have shown that malnutrition in hospitalized patients is more common than previously realized—perhaps as high as 40%. This can stem from the patients' various diseases, as well as any inadequate dietary habits that they exhibited before hospitalization. Either way, such incidents of malnutrition are particularly serious beause they may lead to an array of nutrition-associated complications including respiratory failure, infection, poor wound healing, phlebitis, pulmonary embolism, and fistula formation.

An optimal nutritional status, therefore, is an absolute necessity for the chronically ill, the surgical, or the traumatized patients who already are struggling to regain their health. And nutritional assessment has become an increasingly important tool that can be used by the practitioner in the fight to lower the incidence of these nutrition-associated complications.

The clinician who assesses the nutritional status of a hospitalized patient should do so at various intervals during the hospital stay in order to determine the occurrence and/or severity of malnutrition. The clinician should take serial measurements (in 10- to 14-day intervals) to gain a dynamic sense of the patient's progress and his or her response to medical and nutritional therapies. There are several preliminary cues that suggest suboptimal nutritional status, and particular attention must be paid to the patient's diet and psychological state.

Special Considerations: Case History

It is essential in a hospital practice to identify the high-risk patient. If one of the following factors is present, there is a strong likelihood of malnutrition. On the other hand, the absence of these factors does not automatically ensure that the patient is not malnourished.

The criteria for determining malnutrition risk include:

Is the patient grossly overweight (120% of standard)?
  The risk comes from overlooking protein and calorie requirements in the ill, obese patient.
Is the patient grossly underweight (height/weight less than 80% of standard)?
Has there been a recent loss of 10% or more of bodily weight?
Is the patient an alcoholic?
Is the patient anorexic (can be caused by pain, malignancy, or psychological factors)?
Has the patient been without food for more than 10 days while on intravenous solution?
Does the patient have:
  Malabsorption syndromes
  Short gut fistula
Is the patient on renal analysis?
Does the patient have increased metabolic needs due to:
  Excessive burns
  Infection
  Trauma

Surgery
Protracted fever
Pneumonia
Pregnancy
Obesity
Cachexia
Sepsis
Has the patient experienced:
Intestinal obstruction
Nausea
Vomiting
Acute or chronic blood loss
Diarrhea
Weakness
When did the patient's symptoms begin?
Have there been previous hospitalizations?
What is the patient's medical history?
What is the family medical history?

Special Considerations: Dietary History

What was the patient's prehospital dietary evaluation?
Does the patient presently eat what is on the hospital tray?

Special Considerations: Physical Examination

Muscle wasting
Gingivitis
Delayed wound healing
Decreased tensile strength of wounds
Glossitis
Dermatitis
Petechiae
Ecchymoses
Peripheral neuropathy
Cheilosis
Edema
Pallor
Poor skin turgor
Dry skin
Dry mucous membranes
Koilonychia
Tachycardia
Hypogleusia
Dysgeusia
Tremor
Hyperactive deep reflexes
Disorientation
Ataxia
Sunken fontanel (infants)

Special Considerations: Anthropometric Measurements

Several studies have shown that protein-calorie malnutrition of various degrees is found in 25–50% of all medical and surgical patients who have been hospitalized for at least 2 weeks. Because protein-calorie malnutrition has a direct bearing on patient mortality, the clinician must be very aware of the bodily changes associated with its development.

Clinical signs to watch for include:

Weight loss of 10% or more (indicative of impending protein-calorie malnutrition)

Weight loss of 10% or more in a 2-week period when no infection is present (probably a problem of fluid balance rather than loss of either adipose tissue or lean body mass)

Weight loss of 10% or more in a 1- to 3-month period (indicates loss of both adipose tissue and lean body mass and the beginnings of protein-calorie malnutrition)

The clinician should be aware that starvation alone does not cause high mortality rates until a 40% weight loss has occurred. However, a weight loss in combination with illness or injury does result in a high death risk after only a 25% weight loss.

The following tests should be used to evaluate loss of body mass:

Height
Hospitalized weight
Usual weight
Triceps subscapular skinfold
Midupper arm circumference
Midupper arm area

Special Considerations: Drug-Nutrient Interactions

What is the patient's drug history?
Is the patient on any of the following drugs:
  Steroids
  Antitumor agents
  Immunosuppressants
  Antibiotics

Special Considerations: Laboratory Testing

If any of the above criteria indicate possible malnutrition, the practitioner should order several biochemical tests to measure protein storage values, give information on visceral protein status, and help predict immune competency. Variables that should be assessed include:

Serum albumin
Total iron-binding capacity (TIBC)
Serum transferrin
Serum thyroxine-binding prealbumin
White blood cell count
Lymphocytes as a percentage of white blood cell count
Total lymphocyte count
24-hour urinary creatine
Creatinine-height index (CHI)
Skin test results

Information on the various tests neccesary to obtain these variables is offered below:

Serum albumin and transferrin

Plasma protein decreases as the body loses protein stores. Both serum albumin and serum transferrin levels can be measured as an estimate of visceral protein status (see Table 6.2). However, these levels may be altered by organ failure, particularly in severe liver diseases, severe or acute renal disease, and congestive heart failure. The clinician must then evaluate the patient using dietary and medical history plus total nutritional assessment to identify the type and degree of protein-calorie malnutrition.

Creatinine-height index (CHI)

This can be used to measure lean body mass or metabolically active tissue. It also has been shown:

1. To be a more sensitive instrument for measuring the body's nutritional status in malnourished surgical patients than other measurements.
2. That 24-hour creatine excretion, basal oxygen use, and lean body mass are correlated.
3. Another advantage of using these measurements is that fluid retention does not alter a low CHI even when body weight is affected.
4. One disadvantage, however, is that it is necessary to take a 24-hour urine collection for best results.

To measure CHI, the following formula can be utilized:

$$CHI = \frac{\text{Measured Urinary Creatine}}{\text{Ideal Urinary Creatine}} \times 100$$

For example, the normal urinary creatine for a man of 180.3 cm is 1642 mg per day (see Table 6.3). If the actual output were 1300 mg, the CHI would be:

$$\frac{1300}{1642} \times 100 \text{ or } 79.17\% \text{ of normal}$$

Immune competency

The immune status of the patient must be evaluated to gain an accurate picture of his or her response to illness. Cell-mediated immunity is necessary for the host's defense against infection. When this is decreased, there is a corresponding increase in mortality from infectious diseases, especially in average surgical patients. Skin tests can be used to measure cellular immunity with the following antigens:

Candida
Streptokinase-streptodornase
Mumps

Assessing total lymphocyte count

Moderate or severe totals can be measured by use of Table 6.4.

Table 6.2.
Serum Assessments and Malnutrition[a]

The type and degree of a patient's protein-calorie malnutrition can be determined with the help of a measurement of serum albumin and serum transferrin levels.

	Serum Albumin (gm/100ml)	Serum Transferrin (mg/100ml)
Mild	3.1–3.5	150–175
Moderate	2.1–3.0	100–150
Severe	<2.1	<100

[a] From Blackburn GL, Thornton PA. Nutritional assessment of the hospitalized patient. Med Clin North Am 1979;63(5):1103–15.

Table 6.3.
Ideal Urinary Creatinine Values
Values listed herein can be used by the clinician to determine a creatinine-height index measurement of lean body mass or metabolically active tissue.

Men[a]		Women[b]	
Height (cm)	Ideal Creatinine (mg)	Height (cm)	Ideal Creatinine (mg)
157.5	1288	147.3	830
160.0	1325	149.9	851
162.6	1359	152.4	875
165.1	1380	154.9	900
167.6	1420	157.5	925
170.2	1467	160.0	949
172.7	1513	162.6	977
175.3	1555	165.1	1006
177.8	1596	167.6	1044
180.3	1642	170.2	1076
182.9	1691	172.7	1109
185.4	1739	175.3	1141
188.0	1785	177.8	1174
190.5	1831	180.3	1206
193.0	1891	182.9	1240

[a]Creatinine coefficient (men) = 23 mg/kg of ideal body weight.
[b]Creatinine coefficient (women) = 18 mg/kg of ideal body weight.

Table 6.4.
Malnutrition and Immune Competency
The assessment of a patient's total lymphocyte count—accomplished with the assistance of this chart—is an important test when previous measurements indicate malnutrition might be present.

Total	Lymphocyte Count	Skin Test
Moderate	800–1200	5–10
Severe (Kwashiorkor-like)	<800	<5 mm.

Adverse Hospital Practices

In addition to the positive steps mentioned above to help the clinician identify malnutrition in hospitalized patients, there are several practices—if omitted—that can have an adverse impact on nutritional status. These include:
Failure to record at 10- to 14-day intervals the patient's:

Weight
Height
Triceps skinfold
Serum albumin and transferrin
  Creatine-height index
  Lymphocyte count
  Cellular immunity
Prolonged use of intravenous fluids
Withholding of meals due to diagnostic testing

Failure to notice if the patient does not eat food on his tray

Maintaining nothing-by-mouth status for prolonged periods

Failure to recognize increased nutritional needs from illness, injury, or growth

Surgery without prior assessment of nutritional status

Lack of nutritional support after surgery

Failure to recognize the importance of nutrition and its relation to the immune system

Delay of nutritional support until severe depletion occurs until severe depletion occurs

Suggested Readings

Childhood and Adolescence

Ament ME. Malabsorption syndromes in infancy and childhood. J Pediatr 1972;81:685–687.

Barltrop D, Burland W, eds. Mineral metabolism in pediatrics. Philadelphia: FA Davis Co., 1989.

Bayless TM, Paige DM. Lactose intolerance and milk drinking habits. Gastroenterology 1971;60:605.

Beal VA, Meyers AJ. Iron intake, hemoglobin and physical growth during the first two years of life. Pediatrics 1962;30:518.

Burman D. Adolescent nutrition. Practitioner 1979;222:615–623.

Coates TJ, Thoreson CE. Treating obesity in children and adolescents: a review. Am J Pub Health 1978;68:143–151.

Coble YD. Zinc levels and blood enzyme activities in Egyptian male subjects with retarded growth and sexual development. Am J Clin Nutr 1966;19:415.

Cockburn F. Neonatal convulsions associated with primary disturbances of calcium, phosphorus and magnesium metabolism. Arch Dis Child 1973;48:99.

Crispin S. Nutritional status of preschool children II: anthropometric measurements and interrelationships. Am J Clin Nutr 1968;21:1280.

Dobbing J. Cellular growth of the brain: infant vulnerability. Pediatrics 1975;55:2–6.

Fomon SJ, ed. Infant nutrition. 2nd ed. Philadelphia: WB Saunders Company, 1974.

Fomon SJ. A pediatrician looks at early nutrition. Bull NY Acad Med 1971;47:569.

Gyorgy P. The uniqueness of human milk: biochemical aspects. Am J Clin Nutr 1971;24:970.

Hambridge K. Low levels of zinc in hair, anorexia, poor growth and hypogeusia in children. Pediatr Res 1972;6:868.

Hampton MC. Caloric and nutrient intake of teenagers. J Am Diet Assoc 1967;50:385.

Harris I, Wilkinson AW. Magnesium depletion in children Lancet 1971;2:735.

Heald FP. Adolescent nutrition. Med Clin North Amer 1975;59:1329–1336.

Hodges RE, Krehl WA. Nutritional status of teenagers in Iowa. Am J Clin Nutr 1965;17:262–275.

Huenemann RL. Environmental factors associated with preschool obesity. II: obesity and food practices of children at successive age levels. J Am Diet Assoc 1974;64:489.

Huenemann RL. Teenage nutrition and physique. Springfield, Illinois: CC Thomas, 1974.

Krause MV, Mahan LK. Food, nutrition, and diet therapy: a textbook of nutritional care. 7th ed. Philadelphia: WB Saunders Company, 1984.

Lewin PK. Iatrogenic rickets in low-birth weight infants. J Pediatr 1971;78:207.

McKigney JI, Munro HN, eds., Nutrient requirements in adolescence. Cambridge, Massachusetts: MIT Press, 1976.

McWhirter WR. Plasma tocopherol in infants and children. Acta Paediatr Scand 1975;65:446.

Patterson L. Dietary intake and physical development of Phoenix area children. J Am Diet Assoc 1971;59:106.

Pipes PL. Nutrition in infancy and childhood. St Louis: CV Mosby Co., 1977.

Price NO, Bunce GE. Copper, magnesium and zinc balance in preadolescent girls. Am J Clin Nutr 1970;23:258.

Schlage C, Wortberg B. Zinc in the diet of healthy preschool and school children. Acta Pediatr Scand 1972;61:421.

Shils ME, Young VR, eds. Modern nutrition in health and disease. 7th ed. Philadelphia: Lea & Febinger, 1988.

Simoons FJ, Johnson JD. Perspective on milk-drinking and malabsorption of lactose. Pediatrics 1977;59:98–109.

Suskind RB. Pediatric nutrition. New York: Raven Press, 1981.

Tanner JM. Growth and maturation during adolescence. Nutr Rev 1981;39(2):43–55.

Tsang RC. Oh W. Neonatal hypocalcemia in low birth weight infants. Pediatrics 1970;85:773.

Wait B, Blair R. Energy intake of well nourished children and adolescents. Am J Clin Nutr 1969;22:1383.

Williams S. Handbook of maternal and infant nutrition. Berkeley, California: SWR Productions, Inc, 1976.

Pregnancy

Abrams J, Aponte GE. The leg cramp syndrome during pregnancy: the relationship to calcium and phosphorus metabolism. Am J Obstet Gynecol 1958;76:32.

Alperin JB. Haggard ME. Folic acid, pregnancy and abruptio placentae. Am J Clin Nutr 1969;22:1354.

Barnes RH. Dual role of environmental deprivation and malnutrition in retarding intellectual development. Am J Clin Nutr 1976;29:912.

Bergner L, Susser MW. Low birth weight and prenatal nutrition: an interpretive review. Pediatrics 1970;46:946.

Bernhardt IR, Dorsey DJ. Hypervitaminosis A and congenital renal anomalies in a human infant. Obstet Gynecol 1974;43:750.

Cleary RE, Lumeng L. Maternal and fetal plasma levels of pyridoxal phosphate at term: adequacy of vitamin B₆ supplementation during pregnancy. Am J Obstet Gynecol 1970;121:25.

Cohenour SH, Calloway DW. Blood, urine and dietary pantothenic acid levels of pregnant teenagers. Am J Clin Nutr 1972;25:512.

Committee on Maternal Nutrition, Food and Nutrition Board. Maternal nutrition and the course of pregnancy. Washington, DC: National Academy of Sciences, 1970.

Committee on Nutrition. Breast feeding. Pediatrics 1978;62:591–601.

Deeuw NK, Lowenstein L. Iron deficiency and hydremia in normal pregnancy. Medicine 1966;45:291.

Gal I, Sharman IM. Vitamin A in relation to human malformations. In: Woolam, DH, ed. Advances in teratology, Vol 5. New York: Academic Press, 1972.

Grant JA, Heald FP. Complications of adolescent pregnancy: survey of the literature on fetal outcome in adolescence. Clin Pediatr 1972;11:567–70.

Heller S, Salked RM. Riboflavin status in pregnancy. Am J Clin Nutr 1974;27:1225.

Hunscher HA, Tompkins WT. The influence of maternal nutrition on the immediate and long-term outcome of pregnancy. Clin Obstet Gynecol 1970;13:130–44.

Kaminetzky HA, Baker H. Micronutrients in pregnancy. Clin Obstet Gynecol 1977;20:363–80.

Krause MV, Mahan LK. Food, nutrition, and diet therapy: a textbook of nutritional care. 7th ed. Philadelphia: WB Saunders Company, 1984.

Metcoff J. Maternal leukocyte metabolism in fetal malnutrition: nutrition and malnutrition, identification and measurement. Adv Exp Med Biol 1974;49:73–118.

Lindheimer MD, Katz AI. Sodium and diuretics in pregnancy. N Engl J Med 1973;288:891.

Lund CJ, Donovan JC. Blood volume during pregnancy: significance of plasma and red cell volumes. Am J Obstet Gynecol 1967;98:393.

Pike R. Further evidence of deleterious effects produced by sodium restriction during pregnancy. Am J Clin Nutr 1970;23:883.

Pitkin RM. Calcium metabolism in pregnancy: a review. Am J Obstet Gynecol 1975;121:724–37.

Pitkin RM. Nutritional support in obstetrics and gynecology. Clin Obstet Gynecol 1976;19:489–513.

Rosso P. Maternal nutrition, nutrient exchange and fetal growth. In: Winick M, ed. Nutritional disorders of American women. New York: John Wiley and Sons, 1977.

Shils ME, Young VR, eds. Modern nutrition in health and disease. 7th ed. Philadelphia: Lea & Febinger, 1988.

Wichelow MJ. Caloric requirements for successful breast feeding. Arch Dis Child 1975;50:669.

Widdowson EM. Prenatal nutrition. Ann NY Acad Sci 1977;300:188–189.

Worthington BS, Vermeersch J, Williams SR. Nutrition in pregnancy and lactation. St Louis: CV Mosby Co., 1977.

Obesity and Exercise

Bray G. The obese patient. Philadelphia: WB Saunders Co., 1976.

Bray G. Types of human obesity—a system of classification. Obesity Bariatr Med 1973;2:147.

Coates TJ, Thoreson CE. Treating obesity in children and adolescents: a review. Am J Pub Health 1978;68:143–151.

Crawford PB, Hankin JH. Environmental factors associated with preschool obesity. III: dietary intakes, eating patterns, and anthropometric measurements. J Am Diet Assoc 1978;72:589–595.

Escott-Stump, S. Nutrition and diagnosis-related care. 2nd ed. Philadelphia: Lea & Febiger, 1988.

Heald FP. Treatment of obesity in adolescence. Postgrad Med 1972;51:109.

Krause MV, Mahan LK. Food, nutrition, and diet therapy: a textbook of nutritional care. 7th ed. Philadelphia: W.B. Saunders Company, 1984.

Mayer J. Obesity in adolescence. Med Clin North Am 1965;49:421.

Shils ME, Young VR, eds. Modern nutrition in health and disease. 7th ed. Philadelphia: Lea & Febinger, 1988.

Spargo JA, Heald F. Adolescent obesity. Nutr Today 1966;1:2–9.

Weinsier RL, Fuchs RJ. Body fat: its relationship to coronary heart disease, blood pressure, lipids and other risk factors measured in a large male population. Am J Med 1976;61:815.

Winick M. (ed.) Childhood obesity. New York: John Wiley and Sons, 1975.

Anorexia Nervosa

Agras WS, Barlow HN. Behavior modification of anorexia nervosa. Arch Gen Psychiatry 1974;30:279.

Beaumont PJ. Anorexia nervosa in male subjects. Psychother Psychosom 1970;18:365.

Bruch H. Anorexia nervosa. Nutr Today 1978;13:14–18.

Bruch H. Eating disorders: obesity, anorexia nervosa, and the person within. New York: Basic Books, 1973.

Halmi KA. Anorexia nervosa: demographic and clinical features in 94 cases. Psychosom Med 1974;36:18.

Hurd II HP, Palumbo PJ. Hypothalmic-endocrine dysfunction in anorexia nervosa. Mayo Clin Proc 1977;52:711–716.

Katz JL, Weiner H. A functional anterior hypothalmic defect in primary anorexia nervosa. Psychosom Med 1975;37:103–105.

Krause MV, Mahan LK. Food, nutrition, and diet therapy: a textbook of nutritional care. 7th ed. Philadelphia: WB Saunders Company, 1984.

Lupton M, Simon L. Minireview: biological aspects of anorexia nervosa. Life Sci 1976;18:1341.

Maxmen JS, Silberfarb PM. Anorexia nervosa. J Am Med Assoc 1974;229:801.

Schleimer K. Anorexia nervosa. Nutr Rev 1981;39(2):99–103.

Shils ME, Young VR, eds. Modern nutrition in health and disease. 7th ed. Philadelphia: Lea & Febinger, 1988.

Theander S. Anorexia nervosa. A psychiatric investigation of 94 female patients. Acta Psychiatr Scand 1970;(suppl): 214.

Athletic Performance

Aloai JF. Exercise and skeletal health. J Am Geriatrics Soc 1981;29:104.

Bernard RJ. Effects of an intensive exercise and nutrition program on patients with coronary artery disease: five-year follow-up. J Cardiac Rehab 1983;3:183.

Bentivegna A. Diet, fitness and athletic performance. Phys Sportsmed 1979;7(10):99.

Clement DB, Sawchuk LL. Iron status and sports performance. Sports Med 1984;1:65.

Costill DL, Miller JM. Nutrition for endurance sport: carbohydrate and fluid balance. Int J Sports Med 1982;306:895.

Escott-Stump, S. Nutrition and diagnosis-related care. 2nd ed. Philadelphia: Lea & Febiger, 1988.

Felig P, Wahren J. Fuel homeostasis in exercise. N Engl J Med 1975;293:1078.

Konstantin N. Effects of dieting and exercise on lean body mass, oxygen uptake, and strength. Med Sci Sports Exerc 1985;17:466.

Krause MV, Mahan LK. Food, nutrition, and diet therapy: a textbook of nutritional care. 7th ed. Philadelphia: WB Saunders Company, 1984.

McArdle WD, Katch FI, Katch VL. Exercise physiology: energy, nutrition, and human performance. 2nd ed. Philadelphia: Lea & Febiger, 1986.

Sady SP, Freedson PS. Body composition and structural comparisons of female and male athletes. Clin Sports Med 1984;3:755.

Smith EL. Exercise for prevention of osteoporosis: a review. Phys Sportsmed 1982;10(3):72.

Van Dam B. Vitamins and sports. Br J Sports Med 1978;12:74.

Werblow JA. Nutritional knowledge, attitudes, and food patterns of women athletes. J Am Diet Assoc 1978;73:242.

Wilmore JH. Body composition. Phys Sportsmed 1986;3:144–162.

Musculoskeletal System

Alfano MC. Controversies, perspectives, and clinical implications of nutrition in periodontal diseases. Dent Clin North Am 1976;20:519.

Escott-Stump, S. Nutrition and diagnosis-related care. 2nd ed. Philadelphia: Lea & Febiger, 1988.

Freeland JH, Cousins RJ, Schwartz R. Relationship of mineral status and intake to periodontal disease. Am J Clin Nutr 1976;29:745.

Heany RP. Calcium nutrition and bone health in the elderly. Am J Clin Nutr 1982;36:986.

Krause MV, Mahan LK. Food, nutrition, and diet therapy: a textbook of nutritional care. 7th ed. Philadelphia: WB Saunders Company, 1984.

Maclachan MJ, Rodnan GP. Effects of food, fast and alcohol on serum uric acid and acute attacks of gout. Am J Med 1967;42:38.

Newbrun E. Sugar and dental caries: a review of human studies. Science (Wash DC) 1982;217:418.

Shils ME, Young VR, eds. Modern nutrition in health and disease. 7th ed. Philadelphia: Lea & Febinger, 1988.

Food Allergies

Bock SA. Food sensitivity: a critical review and practical approach. Am J Dis Child 1980;134:973.

Brostoff J, Challacombe SJ, eds. Food allergy. Clin Immunol Allergy 1982;2:1–260.

Heiner DC, ed. Food allergy. Clin Rev Allergy 1984;2:1–93.

Krause MV, Mahan LK. Food, nutrition, and diet therapy: a textbook of nutritional care. 7th ed. Philadelphia: W.B. Saunders Company, 1984.

May CD, Block SA. A modern clinical approach to food hypersensitivity. Allergy 1978;33:166–188.

McCarthy EP, Frick OL. Food sensitivity: keys to diagnosis. J Pediatr 1983;102:645.

Shils ME, Young VR, eds. Modern nutrition in health and disease. 7th ed. Philadelphia: Lea & Febinger, 1988.

Anemias

Beissner R. Clinical assessment of anemia. Postgrad Med 1986;80:83.

Dallkman PR. Iron deficiency: diagnosis and treatment. West J Med 1981;134:496.

Escott-Stump, S. Nutrition and diagnosis-related care. 2nd ed. Philadelphia: Lea & Febiger, 1988.

Herbert, V. The nutritional anemias. Hosp Prac 1980;15:65–89.

Krause MV, Mahan LK. Food, nutrition, and diet therapy: a textbook of nutritional care. 7th ed. Philadelphia: WB Saunders Company, 1984.

Simko MD, Cowell C, Gilbride JA. Nutrition assessment: a comprehensive guide for planning intervention. Rockville, Maryland: Aspen Publishers Inc, 1984.

Immune System

Arbeter A, Echeverri L. Nutrition and infection. Fed Proc 1971;30:1421–28.

Braun W, Ungar J. "Non-specific" factors influencing host resistance. Basel: S Karger, 1973.

Dionigi P, Dionigi R. Nutritional and immunological evaluations in cancer patients: surgical infections. J Parent Ent Nutr 1980;44(4):351–356.

Dreizen S. Nutrition and the immune response—a review. Int J Vit Nutr Res 1979;49:220–228.

Flynn A. Zinc deficiency with altered adreno-cortical function and its relation to delayed healing. Lancet 1973;1:789–791.

Hodges RE. Nutrition in relation to infection. Med Clin North Am 1964;48:1153–1167.

Krause MV, Mahan LK. Food, nutrition, and diet therapy: a textbook of nutritional care. 7th ed. Philadelphia: WB Saunders Company, 1984.

Reddy V, Srikantia SG. Nutrition and the immune response. Indian J Med Res 1978;68(suppl.):48–57.

Schonland M. Depression of immunity in protein-calorie malnutrition: a post-mortem study. J Trop Pediatr 1972;18:217–224.

Scrimshaw NS, Taylor CE. Interactions of nutrition and infection (monograph 57). Geneva: WHO, 1968.

Shils ME, Young VR, eds. Modern nutrition in health and disease. 7th ed. Philadelphia: Lea & Febinger, 1988.

Smythe PM, Schonland M. Thymolymphatic deficiency and depression of cell mediated immunity in protein-calorie malnutrition. Lancet 1971;2:939–943.

Suskind RM, ed. Malnutrition and the immune response. New York: Raven Press, 1977.

Cardiovascular Disease

Castelli WP, Garrison RJ, Wilson PW, et al. Incidence of coronary heart disease and lipoprotein cholesterol level: the Framingham study. JAMA 1986;256(20):2835–2838.

Dawberg TR. Eggs, serum cholesterol and coronary heart disease. Am J Clin Nutr 1982;36:617.

Escott-Stump, S. Nutrition and diagnosis-related care. 2nd ed. Philadelphia: Lea & Febiger, 1988.

Glueck CJ. Dietary fat and arteriosclerosis. Am J Clin Nutr 1979;32:2703.

Gordon T. High-density lipoprotein as a protective factor against coronary artery disease: the Framingham study. Am J Med 1977;62:707–714.

Harper AE. Coronary heart disease: an epidemic related to diet. Am J Clin nutr 1983;37:669.

Johnson BG, Nilsson-Ehle P. Alcohol consumption and high density lipoprotein. N Engl J Med 1978;298:633.

Kaplan NM. Mild hypertension: when and how to treat. Arch Intern Med 1983;143:255.

Krause MV, Mahan LK. Food, nutrition, and diet therapy: a textbook of nutritional care. 7th ed. Philadelphia: WB Saunders Company, 1984.

LaCroix AZ, Mead LA, Liang KY, et al. Coffee consumption and the incidence of coronary heart disease. N Engl J Med 1986;315(16)977–982.

Lavie CJ, Squires W, Gau GT. What is the role of fish and fish oils in the primary and secondary prevention of cardiovascular disease? J Cardiopul Rehabil 1987;7:526–533.

Levy RI, Moskowitz J. Cardiovascular research: decades of progress, a decade of promise. Science (Wash DC) 1982;217:121.

MacMahon S. Alcohol consumption and hypertension. Hypertension 1987;9(2):111–121.

O'Keefe Jr. JH, Lavie CJ, O'Keefe JO. Dietary prevention of coronary heart diease: how to help patients modify eating habits and reduce cholesterol. Postgrad Med 1989;6:243–261.

Stamler J. Diet and coronary heart disease. Biometrics 1982;38(supp):95.

Geriatrics and Degenerative Disease

Butler RN, Lewis MI. Concise handbook on aging. St. Louis: CV Mosby Co, 1977.

Caird FI, Judge TG. Assessment of the elderly patient (1st ed) New York: Lippincott, 1974.

Escott-Stump, S. Nutrition and diagnosis-related care. 2nd ed. Philadelphia: Lea & Febiger, 1988.

Jordan VE. Protein status of the elderly as measured by dietary intake, hair tissue and serum albumin. Am J Clin Nutr 1976;29:522.

Justice CL, Hive JM. Dietary intakes and nutritional status of elderly patients. J Am Diet Assoc 1974;65:639.

Krause MV, Mahan LK. Food, nutrition, and diet therapy: a textbook of nutritional care. 7th ed. Philadelphia: WB Saunders Company, 1984.

McGandy RB, Barrows Jr CH. Nutrient intakes and energy expenditure in men of different ages. J Gerontol 1966;21:581–587.

Munro HN. Protein metabolism in the elderly. Postgrad Med 1978;63:143.

Novak LP. Aging, total body potassium, fat-free mass, and cell mass in males and females between ages 18 and 85 years. J Gerontol 1972;27:438–443.

Rockstein M, Sussman ML, eds. Nutrition, longevity and aging. New York: Academic Press, 1976.

Shils ME, Young VR, eds. Modern nutrition in health and disease. 7th ed. Philadelphia: Lea & Febinger, 1988.

Sullivan JF, Blotcky AJ. Serum levels of selenium, calcium, copper, magnesium, manganese and zinc in various human diseases. J Nutr 1979;109:1432–1437.

Timiras PS. Developmental psysiology and aging. New York: Macmillan, 1972.

Vir SC, Love AH. Nutritional evaluation of B groups of vitamins in institutionalized aged. Int J Vit Nutr Res 1977;47:211–218.

Winick M, ed. Nutrition and aging. New York: John Wiley and Sons, 1976.

The Hospitalized Patient

Bistrian BR, Blackburn GL. Prevalence of malnutrition in general medical patients. JAMA 1976;235:1567–1570.

Bistrian BR, Blackburn GL. Protein status of general surgical patients. JAMA 1974;230:858–860.

Blackburn GL. Nutritional assessment and support during infection. Am J Clin Nutr 1977;30:1493–1497.

Blackburn GL, Thornton PA. Nutritional assessment of the hospitalized patient. Med Clin N Am 1979;63(5):1103–1116.

Blackburn GL, Bistrian BR. Nutritional and metabolic assessment of the hospitalized patient. J Parent Ent Nutr 1977;1:11–22.

Blackburn GL, Bistrian BS. Manual for nutritional-metabolic assessment of the hospitalized patient. New England Deaconness Hospital, Boston, Massachusets, 1976.

Bollet JB, Owens S. Evaluation of nutrition status of selected hospitalized patients. Am J Clin Nutr 1973;26:931.

Butterworth CE. The skeleton in the hospital closet. Nutr Today 1974;9:4.

Butterworth CE, Blackburn GL. Hospital malnutrition and how to assess the nutritional status of a patient. Nutr Today 1975;10(2):March/April.

Detsky AS, Baker JP, Mendelson RA, et al. Evaluating the accuracy of nutritional assessment techniques applied to hospitalized patients: methodology and comparisons. J Parent Ent Nutr 1984;2:153–159.

Krause MV, Mahan LK. Food, nutrition, and diet therapy: a textbook of nutritional care. 7th ed. Philadelphia: WB Saunders Company, 1984.

Law DK, Dudreck SJ. Immunocompetence of patients with protein-calorie malnutrition: the effects of nutrition repletion. Ann Intern Med 1973;79:545–550.

Leevy CM, Cardi L. Incidence and significance of hypovitaminemia in a randomly selected municipal hospital populace. Am J Clin Nutr 1965;17:259.

Merritt RJ, Suskind RM. Nutritional survey of hospitalized pediatric patients. Am J Clin Nutr 1979;32(6):1320–1325.

Newmann CG. Interaction of malnutrition and infection—a neglected clinical concept. Arch Intern Med 1977;370:1364–1365.

Sokal VE. Measurement of delayed skin test responses. N Engl J Med 1975;293:501–502.

Underwood EJ. Trace elements in human and animal nutrition. New York: Academic Press, Inc, 1971.

Weinsier RL, Krumdieck CL, Butterworth Jr. CE. Hospital malnutrition: a prospective evaluation of general medical patients during the course of hospitalization. Am J Clin Nutr 1979;32:418–426.

White RG, Coward WA. Serum-albumin concentration and the onset of kwashiorkor. Lancet 1973;1:63–66.

7

Additional Resources

There is a wide variety of organizations available that offer information to assist the clinician who practices the clinical assessment of nutritional status. These range from national and local associations and groups producing nutritional information, to companies that market hardware and software products specifically for computerized assessments. Some provide patient education materials whereas others produce information that is strictly for use by the practitioner. Addresses and phone numbers for many of these sources are detailed on the following pages; many others can be obtained through these initial contacts.

Health Care Information

National Organizations

Action on Smoking and Health
2013 H Street, N.W.
Washington, D.C. 20006
(202) 658-4310

Administration on Aging
Office of Human Development
U.S. Department of Health and
 Human Services
Washington, D.C. 20201

Agricultural Research Service
Consumer and Food Economics
 Research Division
U.S. Department of Agriculture
Washington, D.C. 20250

American Academy of Pediatrics
1801 Hinman Avenue
Evanston, IL 60201

**American Association for Health,
 Physical Education and Recreation**
1201 Sixteenth Street, N.W.
Washington, D.C. 20016

American Cancer Society
777 Third Avenue
New York, NY 10017

**American College of Obstetricians
 and Gynecologists**
1 East Wacker Drive
Chicago, IL 60601

American Dental Association
211 East Chicago Avenue
Chicago, IL 60611

American Diabetes Association
Publications Department
600 Fifth Avenue
New York, NY 10020

American Dietetic Association
Publications Department
620 North Michigan Avenue
Chicago, IL 60611

American Health Foundation
320 East 43rd Street
New York, NY 10016

American Heart Association
205 East 42nd Street
New York, NY 10017

American Home Economics Association
1600 Twentieth Street, N.W.
Washington, D.C. 20036

American Institute of Baking
Consumer Service Department
400 E. Ontario St.
Chicago, IL 60611

American Medical Association
Order Department
535 North Dearborn Street
Chicago, IL 60610

American Lung Association
1740 Broadway
New York, NY 10019
(212) 315-8700

American Public Health Association
Food and Nutrition Section
1790 Broadway
New York, NY 10019

American Red Cross, Nutritional Education Program
17th and E Streets, N.W.
Washington, D.C. 20006

Arthritis Information Clearinghouse
P.O. Box 9782
Arlington, VA 22209
(703) 558-4999

Association of Heart Patients
P.O. Box 54305
Atlanta, GA 30308
(800) 241-6993

Blue Cross Assocation
840 North Lake Shore Drive
Chicago, IL 60611

Blue Shield Association
211 E. Chicago Avenue
Chicago, IL 60611

Center for Health Promotion and Education
Centers for Disease Control
1600 Clifton Road
Building 1, SSB-249
Atlanta, GA 30333
(404) 329-3492

Center for Science in the Public Interest
1755 S Street, N.W.
Washington, D.C. 20009

Clearinghouse on the Handicapped
400 Maryland Ave., S.W.
3119 Switzer Building
Washington, DC 20202
(202) 245-0080

Extension Service/Home Economics
U.S. Department of Agriculture
Washington, D.C. 20250

Food and Drug Administration
Office of Consumer Affairs
5600 Fishers Lane (HFE-88)
Rockville, MD 20857
(301) 443-3170

Food and Nutrition Information Center
National Agricultural Library Building
Room 304
10301 Baltimore Blvd.
Beltsville, MD 20705
(301) 344-3719

Hemochromatosis Research Foundation
P.O. Box 8569
Albany, NY 12208

High Blood Pressure Information Center
120/80 National Institutes of Health
Bethesda, MD 20892
(703) 558-4880

Iron Overload Disease Association (IOD)
224 Datura Street
Suite 912
West Palm Beach, FL 33401
(305) 659-5616

National Cancer Institute
9000 Rockville Pike
Building 31, Room 10A18
Bethesda, MD 20205
(301) 496-5583

National Center for Health Statistics
Division of Epidemiology and Health Promotion
3700 East-West Highway
Room 2-27
Hyattsville, MD 20782

National Center for Education in Maternal and Child Health
3520 Prospect Street
Ground Floor
Washington, D.C. 20057
(202) 625-8400

National Clearinghouse for Alcohol Information
P.O. Box 2345
Rockville, MD 20852
(301) 468-2600

National Clearinghouse for Family Planning Information
P.O. Box 2225
Rockville, MD 20852
(301) 881-9400

National Clearinghouse for Mental Health Information
Public Inquiries Section
5600 Fishers Lane
Room 15C-05
Rockville, MD 20857
(301) 443-4513

National Dairy Council
111 North Canal Street
Chicago, IL 60606

National Diabetes Information Clearinghouse
Box: NDIC
Bethesda, MD 20892
(301) 468-6344

National Digestive Diseases Education and Information Clearinghouse
1255 23rd St. N.W.
Suite 275
Washington, D.C. 20037

National Health Information Clearinghouse
P.O. Box 1133
Washington, DC 2003-1133
(202) 429-9091

National Institutes of Health
U.S. Department of Health, Education, and Welfare
8600 Rockville Pike
Bethesda, MD 20014

National Interagency Council on Smoking and Health
90 Park Avenue
New York, NY 10019
(212) 599-8200

National Library of Medicine
Literature Search Program
Reference Section
U.S. Department of Education
8600 Rockville Pike
Bethesda, MD 20014

National March of Dimes Foundation
Professional Education Department
P.O. Box 2000
White Plains, NY 10602

National Rehabilitation Information Center
4407 Eighth Street, N.E.
Washington, D.C. 20017-2299
(202) 635-5822

National Research Council
Food and Nutrition Board
2101 Constitution Ave., N.W.
Washington, D.C. 20037

The Nutrition Foundation
489 Fifth Avenue
New York, NY 10017

Nutrition Information and Resource Center
Benedict House
The Pennsylvania State University
University Park, PA 16802
(814) 865-6323

Office of Disease Prevention and Health Prevention
U.S. Department of Health and Human Services
Washington, D.C. 20201

Office on Smoking and Health
Technical Information Center
5600 Fishers Lane
Park Building, Room 116
Rockville, MD 20857
(301) 443-1690

President's Council on Physical Fitness and Sports
400 6th Street, S.W., Suite 3030
Washington, D.C. 20201

Society for Nutrition Education
National Nutrition Education Clearinghouse
2140 Shattuck Avenue
Suite 1110
Berkeley, CA 94704

U.S. Department of Health and Human Services
Office on Smoking and Health
5600 Fishers Lane
Rockville, MD 20857
(202) 443-1575

U.S. National Library of Medicine
Bethesda, MD 20014

Local Organizations

City Health Department
Contacts: check local phone book
Colleges and Universities
Contacts: medicine, nursing, nutrition, public health
County Health Department
Contacts: check local phone book
Medical Centers and Hospitals
Contacts: dietary and/or nutrition departments

State Extension Service/Department of Home Economics
Contacts: check local state college or university
State Health Department
Contacts: check phone book (most likely in state capital)

Computer Information

Selected Software Distributors

AB Software Inc.
Box 3737
Greenville, NC 27834
(919) 752-2556

ABT Associates Inc.
55 Wheeler Street
Cambridge, MA 02138
(617) 492-7100

AGNET
105 Miller Hall
University of Nebraska
Lincoln, NE 68583
(402) 472-1892

Agricultural Communications Center
Ag Science 111
University of Idaho
Moscow, ID 83843
(203) 885-7984

Agricultural Extension Service—EXTEND
University of Minnesota
475 Coffey Hall
1420 Eckles Street
St. Paul, MN 55113
(612) 376-7003

Anjon Systems Inc.
Box 4278
South Bend, IN 46617
(219) 233-6695

Arkansas Department of Education
NET Coordinator
Capitol Mall
Little Rock, AR 72201
(501) 371-2063

Capital Systems Group Inc.
7910 Woodmont Avenue
Suite 208
Bethesda, MD 28014

W.O. Caster, PhD
167 Dawson Hall
Department of Foods and Nutrition
University of Georgia
Athens, GA 30602
(404) 542-2551

clo's-line
Volborg, MT 59351
(406) 784-2280

Colorado State University
Department of Food Science and Nutrition
Cooperative Extension Service

c/o Jennifer E. Anderson
200 Gifford Building
Fort Collins, CO 80523
(303) 491-7334

ComCater International Inc.
65 South Main Street
Pennington, NJ 08534
(609) 737-1540

Computerized Management Systems
1039 Cadiz Drive
Simi, CA 93065
(805) 526-0151

Computerized Nutritional Analysis
21700 76th Avenue, W.
Suite 105
Edmonds, WA 98020
(206) 775-8646

Computrition Inc.
21049 Devonshire Street
Chatsworth, CA 91311
(800) 222-4488, (818) 341-9739

Marc Covitt, Programs "R" Us
199 N. El Camino Real
F-301
Encinitas, CA 92024
(619) 942-7148

DDA (Dietary Data Analysis)
P.O. Box 26
Hamburg, NJ 07419
(201) 764-6677

DEG Software Inc.
11999 Katy Freeway
Suite 150
Houston, TX 77079
(800) 231-0627, (713) 531-6100

Theresa Devriendt
6110 W. 92nd Place
Westminster, CO 80030
(303) 427-9739

Diabetes Research and Training Center
Albert Einstein College of Medicine
1300 Morris Park Avenue
Bronx, NY 10461
(212) 430-4096

Dietware
Box 503
Spring, TX 77383
(713) 440-6943

DINESystems Inc.
2211 Main Street
Building B
Buffalo, NY 14214

Ruth M. Dow, PhD, RD
School of Home Economics
Eastern Illinois University
Charleston, IL 61920
(217) 581-3223

EBNA
Box 34882
Bethesda, MD 20817

EMC Publishing
300 York Avenue
St. Paul, MN 55101
(800) 328-1452

ESHA Research
P.O. Box 13028
Salem, OR 97309
(503) 585-6242

Evryware
1950 Cooley Avenue
6208
Palo Alto, CA 94303
(415) 321-2708

Family Living Education
Cooperative Extension Service
Extended Nutrition Program
202 Wills House
Michigan State University
East Lansing, MI 48824
(517) 353-9102

A. Frashier, D Ph
347 Wauford
Nashville, TN 37211
days: (615) 865-2373, ext. 4522
after 6 p.m.: (615) 331-0167

Eldon Fredericks
Agriculture Communication Service
Ag Ad Building
West Lafayette, IN 47907
(317) 494-8333

Genesee Intermediate S/D
c/o Gloria Bourdon
2413 W. Maple Avenue
Flint, MI 48507
(313) 767-4310

Liane Giambalvo and Katherine O. Musgrave
School of Human Development

University of Maine
Orono, ME 04469
(207) 581-3130

Health Development Inc.
Nutrition Services Division
1165 West Third Avenue
Columbus, OH 43212
(800) 222-4630, (614) 294-2688

Healthpath Associates
68 Olive Street
Chagrin Falls, OH 44022
(216) 247-5298

**HEEF Health Enhancement and
Promotions Company**
Box 546
Ames, IA 50010
(515) 233-3552

A.M. Hills
14504 Deer Ridge Drive, S.E.
Calgary, Alberta
Canada T2J 5W8
(403) 278-0180

HMS Associates
18 Greenway Gables
Minneapolis, MN 55403
(612) 370-0720

Zoe Ann Holmes
Department of Foods and Nutrition
Oregon State University
Corvallis, OR 97331
(503) 754-3561

Intake
Box 555
Port Jefferson Station, NY 11776
(516) 331-1481

**International Publishing and
Software Inc.**
3948 Chesswood Drive
Downsview, Ontario
Canada M3J 2W6
(416) 636-9409

IPC Datadiet
350 N. Lantana
565
Box 3000
Camarillo, CA 93011
(805) 484-1616

Norge W. Jerome, PhD
Community Nutrition Lab, 5030 B
University of Kansas Medical Center

39th and Rainbow
Kansas City, KS 66103
(816) 588-2792

Knossos Inc.
422 Redwood Avenue
Corte Madera, CA 94925
(415) 924-8528

Harriet Kohn
Extension Food and Nutrition
  Specialist
315 Leverton Hall
East Campus, UNL
Lincoln, NE 68583-0808
(402) 472-3717

Lawrence Hall of Science
Math and Computer Education
  Project
University of California
Berkeley, CA 94720
(415) 642-3167

The Learning Seed
21250 Andover Road
Kildeer, IL 60047
(312) 397-4470

Marshfilm Enterprises Inc.
Box 8082
Shawnee Mission, KS 66208
(816) 523-1059

Medical Data Management Systems
7372 Prince Drive
Suite 107
Huntington Beach, CA 92647
(714) 841-5557

Medical Software Systems Company
4812 S.W. Ninth Street
Des Moines, IA 50315
(515) 285-4098

Microcater Systems
22 Blue Hill Road
Amherst, MA 01002
(413) 253-3522

Microcomp
2015 NW Circle Boulevard
Corvallis, OR 97330
(503) 754-0811

Micromedx
187 Gardiners Avenue
Levittown, NY 11756
(516) 735-8979

Minnesota Educational Computing Consortium (MECC)
3490 Lexington Avenue, N.
St. Paul, MN 55112
(612) 481-3500

Pat Munyon
2015 Caminito San Nicholas
La Jolla, CA 92037
(619) 230-6851

Muse Software
347 N. Charles Street
Baltimore, MD 21201
(301) 659-7212

N-Squared Computing
5318 Forest Ridge Road
Silverton, OR 97381
(503) 873-5906

National Dairy Council
6300 N. River Road
Rosemont, IL 60018
(312) 696-1020

NDDA Laboratory
Food and Nutrition
College of Agriculture
Southern Illinois University
Carbondale, IL 62901
(618) 453-5193

NutriMed Inc.
1701 N. Greenville Avenue
Suite 712
Richardson, TX 75081
(214) 669-2465

Nutrition and Diet Services
Chedwah J. Stein, RD, MS
927 S.E. Rimrock Lane
Portland, OR 97222
(503) 654-3583

Nutrition Computer and Statistical Service Inc.
15 Linden Street
Great Neck, NY 11020
(516) 466-8162

Nutrition Consultants Inc.
Box 1513
Norman, OK 73070
(405) 329-7994

Nutrition Design
3406 S.W. Chintimini Avenue
Corvallis, OR 97333
(503) 758-1280

Nutrition Information Systems
Box 1199
Barrington, IL 60010
(312) 934-4874

Nutrition Software
Box 2926
Country Club Hills, IL 60477
(312) 798-1039

The Ohio State University Hospitals
Department of Dietetics
c/o Diane Clapp, MS, RD
410 W. 10th Avenue
Room 158
Columbus, OH 43210
(614) 421-3894

Orange Juice Software Systems
222 S. Washington Avenue
New Richmond, WI 54017
(715) 246-3588

PCD Systems Inc.
163 Main Street
Box 277
Penn Yan, NY 14527-0277
(315) 536-7428

Pennsylvania State University
Nutrition Education Center
University Park, PA 16802
(814) 865-6323

The Pillsbury Company
M/S 3286
Pillsbury Center
Minneapolis, MN 55402
(612) 330-8732

Practical Programs
1104 Aspen Drive
Toms River, NJ 08753

Practocare Inc.
10951 Sorrento Valley Road
Suite II-F
San Diego, CA 92121
(619) 450-0553

Profile Associates
100 Eastowne Drive
Chapel Hill, NC 27514
(919) 967-9400

Public Interest Software
Center for Science in the Public Interest
1501 16th Street, N.W.
Washington, D.C. 20036

(202) 332-9110

RJL Systems Inc.
9930 Whittier
Detroit, MI 48224
(800) 528-4513, (313) 881-2030

Scott, Foresman, and Company
Electronic Publishing Division
1900 East Lake Avenue
Glenview, IL 60025
(312) 729-3000

Sarah H. Short, Phd, EdD, RD
300 Slocum Hall
Syracuse University
Syracuse, NY 13210
(315) 423-2386

SN Services
4659 East Amherst Avenue
Denver, CO 80222
(303) 756-0398

Soft Bite Inc.
Box 1484
East Lansing, MI 48823
(517) 337-1253

The Software Toolworks
15233 Ventura Boulevard
Suite 1118
Sherman Oaks, CA 91403
(818) 986-4855

Sunburst Communications Inc.
39 Washington Avenue
Pleasantville, NY 10570
(800) 431-1934

Super Software Systems Ltd.
San Michele
Beech Hill Road
Hampshire, England GU 35 8DN
(0428) 713050

Suzanne Tenold
Regional Food and Nutrition
  Specialist
Alberta Agricultural Home Economics
Bag Service 1
Airdrie, Alberta
Canada T0M 0B0
(403) 948-5101

Transcontinental Health Data
Marketing Department
1783 Eleventh Street
Hampton, VA 23665
(804) 865-0430

University of Missouri
c/o Loretta Hoover, PhD, RD
Dietetic Education
318 Clark Hall
University of Missouri
Columbia, MO 65211
(314) 882-4136

Viking Inc.
c/o Gregory F. Ludwig, President
910 500 Boulevard
Rice Lake, WI 54868
(715) 234-2680

Selected Hardware/Software Combinations

1. Apple
   Apple Pie
   Calorie Study Programs
   Computerized Simulation of the Use of the
     Diabetic Exchange System
   Cost-Study Program
   The Daily Menu Analyzer
   Dietician
   The Digestive System: The Disappearing
     Dinner
   The DINE System
   Eat For Health
   Eat Smart Nutrition Computer Program
   Eating Machine
   Eats
   Elementary Vol. 13—Nutrition
   The Energy Nutrients: Sources and
     Functions
   Exchange Based Nutritional Analysis
   Fast Food Micro-Guide
   Food Facts

   Food Poisoning, Sanitation and
     Preservation
   The Food Processor
   Health-Aide
   Health Maintenance—Vol. 1: Facts
   Health Maintenance—Vol. 2: Assessment
   Healthy Meal Planner
   Individualized Diet Management
   Nutra-comp
   Nutri-Bytes
   Nutri-Calc
   Nutrient Analysis System (NAS)
   Nutrilizer
   Nutri-Pack
   Nutriplan
   Nutriplanner—1600
   NutriQuest
   Nutrition and the Basic Four Food Groups
   Nutrition Design
   Nutrition Simulation
   Nutrition Tutorial

Nutrition Vol. 1
Nutrition Vol. 2
Nutritionist
Nutritionist II
Simulated Laboratory Experiments: Investigating the Functional Properties of Food
Sodium and You
Weight Planning
What Did You Eat Yesterday?
What I Usually Eat

2. Digital Equipment Corporation (DEC)
Best of Wok Talk
Computer Chef
Nutri 1
Nutri-Calc
Preserv
Softfit
Sports Conditioning for the United States Olympic Training Center

3. Heath/Zenith
Best of Wok Talk
Computer Chef
Nutricom
Nutritionist
Nutritionist II

4. IBM-PC/XT
Best of Wok Talk
CNA (Comprehensive Nutritional Assessment)
Computer Chef
DAS (Dietary Analysis and Assessment System)
Datadiet Nutrient Analysis
Dietary/Food Management System
Evrydiet: A Nutrition and Diet Guide
Exchange Based Nutritional Analysis (EBNA)
456-Dyette
Health-Aide
Healthpath
InShape
Metabolic Status Profile

Nutranal
Nutri-Bytes
Nutri-Calc
Nutrilizer
Nutriplan
Nutriplanner—1600
NutriQuest
Nutrition Design
Nutritional Analysis Assessment Program
Nutritionist
Nutritionist II
PN Support Module
Recipe Scaling
Softfit
Sports Conditioning for the United States Olympic Training Center
Total Parenteral Nutrition Program

5. Kaypro
Best of Wok Talk
Computer Chef
Nutri-Bytes
Nutritionist
Nutritionist II

6. Radio Shack TRS-80
Apple Pie
Compucal
Diet Evaluation
Easycalc
Fast Food Micro-Guide
Food for Thought
Multicalc
NutriBytes
Nutri-Calc
NutriQuest
Nutrition Consult
Nutrition Information Systems
Nutritional Assessment
Recipe Scaling
Softfit
Total Parenteral Nutrition Formulation
What Did You Eat Yesterday?
Xchancalc

Suggested Readings

Adelman MO, Dwyer JT, Woods M, et al. Computerized dietary analysis systems: a comparative view. Continuing Education 1983;4:421-428.

Byrd-Bredbenner C, Pelican S. Software: how do you choose? J Nutr Educ 1984;16:77.

Byrd-Bredbenner C. Computer nutrient analysis software packages: consideration for selection. Nutr Today 1988;5:13-21.

Brown JE, Hover LW, Cross JK. Shopping for computers. Commun Nutr 1982;1(4):18.

Frank GC, Pelican S. Guidelines for selecting a dietary analysis system. Perspectives in Practice 1986;1:72-75.

Frank RC, ed. Directory of food and nutrition information services and resources. Phoenix: Oryx Press, 1984.

Shannon B, Byrd-Bredbenner C, Pelican S. Computers in nutrition education. J Nutr Educ 1984;16:80.

Wheeler LA, Wheeler ML. Review of microcomputer nutrient analysis and menu planning programs. M D Computing 1984;1(2):42.

APPENDIX:

American Chiropractic Association Statement

The American Chiropractic Association has a certificate board known as the American Chiropractic Board of Nutrition. The Board shall prescribe educational standards and other requirements relative to this specialization. They are required to issue certifications, enhance the educational program, survey and evaluate the facilities in which the course offerings are presented, and monitor all course offerings that fall within the areas of their responsibility.

For a chiropractor to be Board Eligible shall mean that he/she has satisfactorily completed the prescribed 300-hour course of a CCE status college in the field of nutrition or a candidate who has satisfied criteria of a residency program in nutrition.

Only persons who have completed the 300-plus hours by a college having status with CCE may be considered.

Doctors classified as Board Eligible must sit for and successfully negotiate an entire battery of examinations leading to the Diplomate status within three years of completion of this program.

Once a candidate has completed all examinations successfully and has satisfied all criteria of the Board, he/she is then certified as a Diplomate of the American Chiropractic Board of Nutrition and may use the D.A.C.B.N. following his/her name.

While it is not necessary for the chiropractic physician to be a member of a state or national organization, it is necessary that within six months following his or her examination the individual must join and be a member in good standing of the American Chiropractic Association and the ACA Council of Nutrition, to be a member of the American Chiropractic College of Nutrition.

INDEX

Page numbers in *italics* denote figures; those followed by "t" denote tables.

in food allergy, 143

in malabsorption/maldigestion, 101–106, 103t

in malnutrition, 158–160, 159t–160t

in musculoskeletal disorders, 141

medication effects on, 71

mineral supplement effects on, 72–73

normal values, 65, 66t–67t

nutritional supplement effects on, 71–73

obese patients, 135–136

patient preparation for, 70–73

pregnant patients, 133

sensitivity vs. nutrient, 65, 68t–69t

utility, 69–70

vitamin supplement effects on, 71–72

Lactic dehydrogenase (LDH), serum

clinical implications, 82–83

in liver disease, 96–98

normal values, 67t

Lactoferrin, nutritional deficiency effects on, 150

Lactose intolerance test, 105

Lange calipers, in skinfold measurement, 50

Larodopa, nutrient interactions with, 124

Laxatives, malabsorption and, 116, 123

LDH (see Lactic dehydrogenase)

LDL (low-density lipoprotein) cholesterol, 152–153, 153t

Lead toxicity, 23–24

Lean body mass, creatinine-height index and, 159, 160t

Lean body weight

bioelectric impedance assessment, 61, 61–63, 63

in reference man/woman, 60

Leg deformities, causes, 29

Length of infants, measurement methods for, 46

Levodopa, food interactions with, 123

Life events indicator, 7–8

Lip disorders, 27, 40

Lipase, serum, normal values, 66t

Lipids (see also Cholesterol; Fat; Triglycerides)

laboratory tests for, 92, 104

sensitivities, 68t

malabsorption, 104

maldigestion, 102

Liver disorders

chronic passive congestion, 97

enlargement, 30

hepatitis, 97–98

hepatocellular disease, 97

hepatoma, 97

metastatic carcinoma, 97

Liver function tests

disease prognosis and, 96

preferred grouping, 96

purposes, 95

selection for specific diagnosis, 95–98

Low-density lipoprotein cholesterol, 152–153, 153t

Lymphocyte count

malnutrition and, 159, 160t

normal values, 67t

Lysozyme, nutritional deficiency effects on, 150

McGaw calipers in skinfold measurement, 51

Magnesium

deficiency, 21–22, 83

effects on laboratory tests, 73

laboratory tests for, 69t, 95

malabsorption, 106

serum

clinical implications, 83

normal values, 66t

toxicity, 22, 83

Malabsorption

calcium, 116–117

carbohydrates, 104–105

causes, 102

drug-related, 116–117

laboratory tests in, 101–106, 103t

lipids, 104

minerals, 105–106

primary, 116–117

protein, 105

secondary, 117

vitamins, 105–106, 116–124

vs. maldigestion, 102–103, 103t

Maldigestion

carbohydrates, 102

laboratory values in, 103, 103t

protein, 102

vs. malabsorption, 102–103, 103t

Malnutrition, protein-calorie

anthropometric measurement in, 157–158

cell-mediated immunity in, 149–150

clinical signs, 157–158

complications from, 156

creatinine-height index and, 159, 160t

iatrogenic, 160–161

immune system and, 159, 160t

in hospitalized patients, 156–161, 159t–160t

laboratory tests for, 158–160, 159t–160t

serum proteins in, 159, 159t

Manganese

deficiency, 20

malabsorption, 106

toxicity, 20

Marasmus, cell-mediated immunity in, 149

Mean cell hemoglobin concentration (MCH), normal values, 67t

Mean cell volume (MCV), normal values, 67t

Memory disorders, causes, 30

Mental disorders, nutritional causes, 30

Mercury toxicity, 24

Metabolism

drugs, nutrient effects on, 112

increased, conditions associated with, 4–5

thyroid function in, 98

Methotrexate, malabsorption and, 117, 122

Methylmalonic acid test, in vitamin B_{12} deficiency, 148

Mineral oil, malabsorption and, 116, 123

Minerals (see also specific mineral, e.g., Copper; Zinc)

effects on laboratory tests, 72–73

in nutritional history, 17–23

laboratory tests for, 95, 106

malabsorption, 106

Mithramycin, calcium malabsorption and, 122

Moon face, causes, 26

Mouth disorders, 27–28, 40

Mucosal disorders, in vitamin deficiency, 149

Muscle(s)

arm

area measurement, 53–55, 54, 56t, 57, 58–59

circumference measurement, 53–55, 54, 55t, 57, 58–59

in reference man/woman, 60

wasting, causes, 29

weakness, causes, 30

Musculoskeletal disorders

causes, 29

special considerations, 139–141

Myoglobin, urine, normal values, 67t

Nails disorders, causes, 28

Nasolabial seborrhea, causes, 26

Nembutal, nutrient interactions with, 124

Neomycin, malabsorption and, 116, 119

Nervous system disorders, causes, 30

Neutron activation in body composition assessment, 60–62

Niacin (vitamin B_3, nicotinic acid)

deficiency, 11–12

in children, 129

mucocutaneous integrity and, 149

physical signs, 40

effects on laboratory tests, 72

laboratory tests for, 68t, 94

malabsorption, 106

toxicity, 12

Niacinamide (see Niacin)

Nitrogen

body, neutron activation assessment, 60–61

in stool

in malabsorption, 105

normal values, 67t

nonprotein, serum, normal values, 66t

Nitrogen balance, normal values, 66t

Nitroglycerin, alcohol interactions with, 122

Nutrient deficiency (see Deficiency)

Nutrient loss, conditions associated with, 5

Nutritional assessment

indications for, ix–x

model for, x, x

summary form for, 4

Obesity

adverse effects, 133–134

definition, 133

malnutrition with, 156

skin disorders in, 28

special considerations, 133–136

Ophthalmoplegia, causes, 27

Oral contraceptives, vitamin/mineral malabsorption and, 123